AF387479

MEDICAL COLLABORATION WITH ARTIFICIAL INTELLIGENCE

A Real-Life Paradigm Shift

Edition: JDH Éditions
77600 Bussy-Saint-Georges. France
Printed by BoD - Books on Demand, Norderstedt, Germany

ISBN: 978-2-38127-179-8
Legal deposit: July 2022

Adnan El Bakri, MD. MSc.

MEDICAL COLLABORATION WITH ARTIFICIAL INTELLIGENCE

A Real-Life Paradigm Shift

JDH Éditions

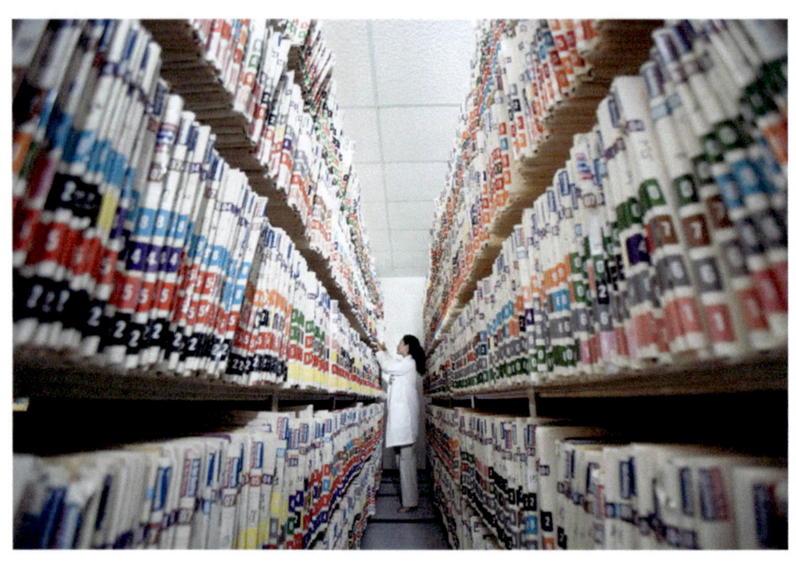

IMAGE SHOWING PATIENT HEALTH RECORD MANAGEMENT AT A HOSPITAL IN FRANCE…

PREFACE

Voluntary Serendipity

It was through a chance meeting during a "Health Hackathon", in the hope of creating the application that was missing from my practice as a surgeon (you are never better served than by yourself), that I met Dr. Adnan El Bakri, then a young urologist in training in Reims.

I was quickly charmed, and his enthusiasm and ambition were obvious. His objective, his project: to free health data from their straitjacket in order to facilitate access to them for patients and caregivers. Better still, he does not only wish to improve on the current rigid and non-interoperable information systems, but also to innovate by exploiting and structuring data to improve the health of all.

He had already started his adventure by creating a major network on e-health, and his company is the first step of an assumed ambition towards the creation of a future world leader, without hesitating to evoke the success of a LinkedIn or a Google of health.
But first, he must complete his studies. I became his thesis supervisor, who linked his research work on the use of artificial intelligence in the monitoring and prediction of kidney cancer. This reinforced his intuition that digital technology and artificial intelligence will be used to improve health.

After many years of hard work, difficulties, disappointments and victories, Adnan El Bakri, a doctor, specialist in e-health and in the structuring of medical data through a new innovative and patented machine learning system, has become a business leader, an influencer in his field, a true inspirational leader. With a remarkable sense of timing, he has developed his platform for medical collaboration aided by artificial intelligence and linked to a digital and universal health passport belonging to the patient, a concept that has become a commercial reality and which makes perfect sense in this era of global pandemics.

Today the solution is ready and operational, and it is this contemporary, original, rare, and essential intellectual path that is communicated in this complete, exceptional and exciting book.

Serendipity can be an accidental sagacity, or the "gift" of making serendipitous discoveries beyond the scope of the initial objective, and this is what I believe my friend Dr. Adnan El Bakri, a forerunner, succeeded in doing, not by chance but by a deep and early conviction.

Professor Michael ATLAN, MD, PhD.
Researcher at INSERM 1148
Lecturer at the Sorbonne Medicine University
Head of the Plastic Surgery Department at Tenon Hospital AP-HP
Paris
Passionate about new technologies in health

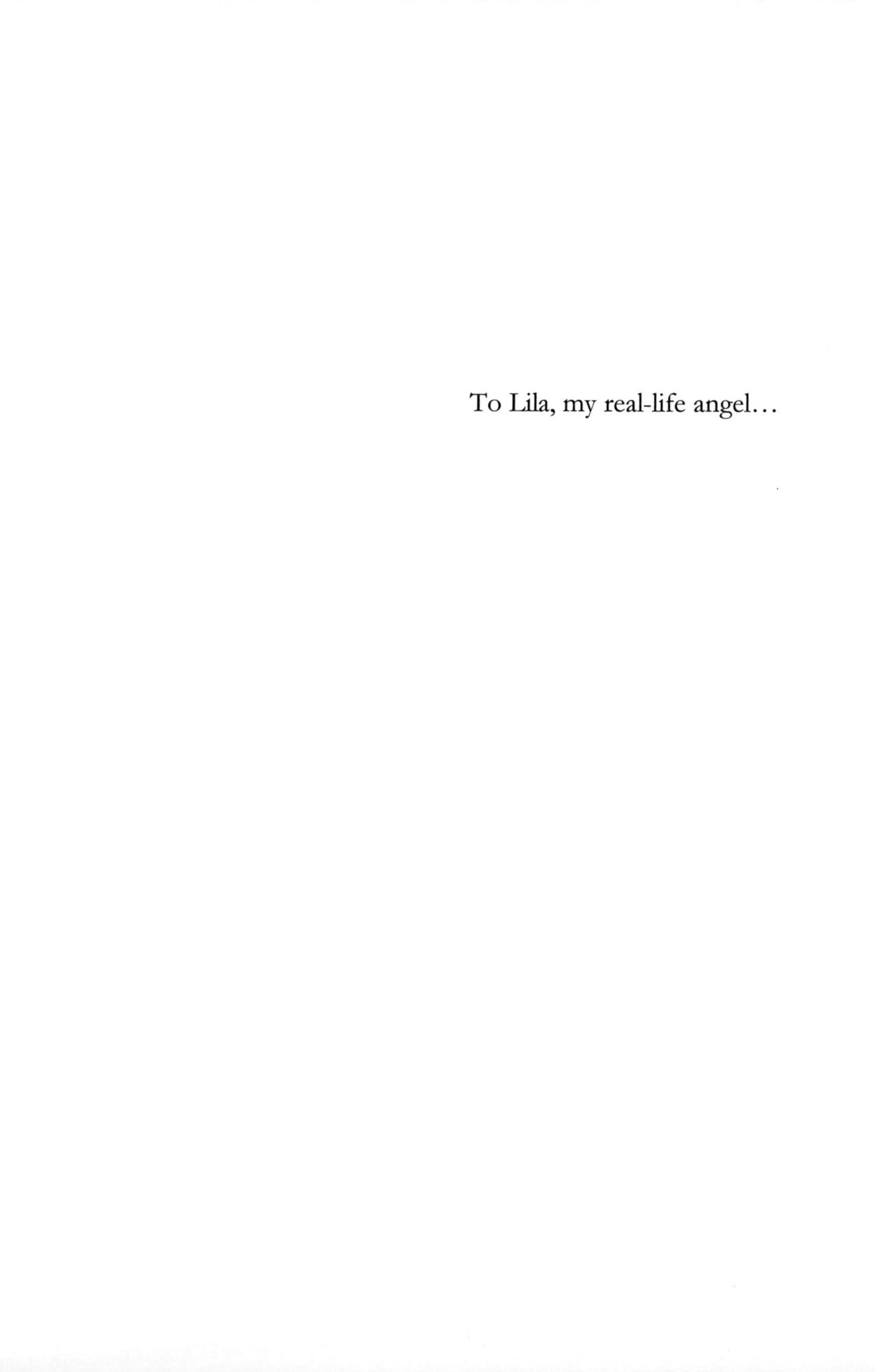

To Lila, my real-life angel…

"An entrepreneur is someone who jumps off a cliff and builds
a plane on the way down."
Reid Hoffmann – Cofounder of LinkedIn

I also dedicate this work to my family, my friends and my wonderful team.

To Jane, Dr. Azzam, Dany, Magedouline, without you this work would not have been feasible!

To Sylvain, Olivier, Marc-Henri, Agathe, Hervé, Dr. Marc, Dr. Charles, Dr. Michael, Dr. François, Dr. Elie, Serge, Pierre, Antoine, Chloé, Lucas, Simon, Mace, Marjorie, Sébastien, Cédric, Dr. Saidé, Dori, Alain, Paolo, and all the ReLyfe Dream Team, Shareholders & Partners…

To Séverine, Thomas, Philippe, Arthur, Dorota, and all their excellent team who made me love lawyers…

To my Reine, for your eagle eye, your sensitivity and strength, your proofreading, you are brilliant, perfect…

To Charlène, for your steadfast support and all we have been through together, I have no regrets…

To my parents, my mum Mona and my dad Maan, to whom I owe everything, my values, my perseverance…

To Ibrahim and Naro, stay positive, better days are on their way…

To Brigitte and Eric, for the good times we have shared together, you are adorable and unforgettable…

To Nadia, for having endured the complexity of all the administrative procedures & bureaucracy…

To Jean-Michel, who is among the wonderful people I encountered who truly believed in me, thank you…

To my family, my sisters Dima, Rayan and Layal, and my little brother Ahmad, and their amazing kids, crazy family…

To my uncle Taha and his cute family…

To my lovely aunts Najwa and Dodi, you made me, I love you dearly…

To Leslie, who became my lucky star and who dreamt of touching the ReLyfe card…

To my aunt Layla, to whom I owe my success and who I miss terribly, bhebbek…
To my elementary school "Rawdet El Zaytoun" in Abou Samra, I remember everything…
To my high school "Saba Zreik" in Tripoli, which built my character, what memories…
To the teachers who passed on the desire to learn, from a very early age…

And to all those who believed in me, but also to those who told me it was impossible!

Lastly, but no doubt there will be those of you I have forgotten, forgive me…
To my country of origin, Lebanon, which is in the midst of a revolution for a better future, and which taught me determination…
To my host country, France, which I thank for giving me the opportunity to succeed…
To you my two dear countries, I now want to contribute to creating the future!

ABSTRACT

E-Health and New Digital Technologies for Medical Data Sharing and Structuring

<u>Introduction</u>
Predictive healthcare requires big data analytics. In practice, however, health information is centralized, inadequately structured, and rarely shared, impeding the application of artificial intelligence. This being the case, the objective was to explore the potential value of e-health in health data sharing and structuring with a view to offering a new, more suitable decentralized technological solution.

<u>Materials and Methods</u>
After a review of the scientific literature, a multicenter case-control study was first conducted using infrared microspectroscopy applied to tumor sections from a retrospective cohort of 100 patients having undergone surgery for kidney cancer and followed for five years. Mathematical clustering was applied to 4 million generated data. This work led to the development of ReLyfe.com, a health card with a unique medical digital identity, connected to a web and mobile platform featuring a new hybrid technological architecture for real-time collaborative sharing and structuring health information. Four years (2016–2019) were dedicated to developing a POC (Proof Of Concept) and then two years (2020-2021) to validating this model in real-life, which required the creation of a company (ReLyfe Group) and the recruitment of engineers. The funding for the research program was provided by Bpifrance, the French Public Investment Bank, healthcare professionals and other private investors.

Results and Discussion

The algorithm used in the first study identified two optical prognostic markers by analyzing the four million data points, demonstrating the predictive potential of a structured big data model produced from a small cohort of patients. However, this lengthy process needs to be validated a posteriori using supervised human classification and so cannot be replicated.

Hence the development of the project for the application of a complete e-health digital platform based on a new, secure hybrid architecture, which allows information to be instantly shared, automatically structured, and decentralized, in a redesigned two-sided economic business model, including electronic traceability of patient consent, facilitating the data's use in research protocols. Although already operational, this model requires more data and long-term application experience and network in order to be democratized in clinical practice.

Conclusion and Perspectives

E-Health and new digital technologies can allow more efficient sharing and better structuring of health data for predictive healthcare. This work paves the way for a paradigm shift with potential future exploitation of real-life health data, providing a continuous supply of information to research departments worldwide, while placing the patient in the center of a better coordinated and connected care pathway everywhere.

Keywords: Digital Health, Medical Collaboration, Care Pathway, Patient Generated Health Data, Personal Health Records, Telemedicine, Big Data, Artificial Intelligence, Renal Cell Carcinoma, Infrared Spectroscopy, Machine Learning, Data Mining, Deep Learning, Optical Character Recognition, Predictive Medicine.

PART ONE

INTRODUCTION

GENERAL INTRODUCTION

Predictive healthcare requires big data analytics. Yet digital developments for healthcare are not keeping pace with new digital technologies. In practice, health information is rarely shared and is inadequately structured, impeding the application of artificial intelligence, particularly in public health. Indeed, the care pathways operate compartmentally, and patients do not have easy access to their data. Given these practical constraints which demonstrate highly centralized architectures, the objective was to explore the potential value of e-health and decentralization in health data sharing and structuring with a view to offering a new technological solution (Figure 1).

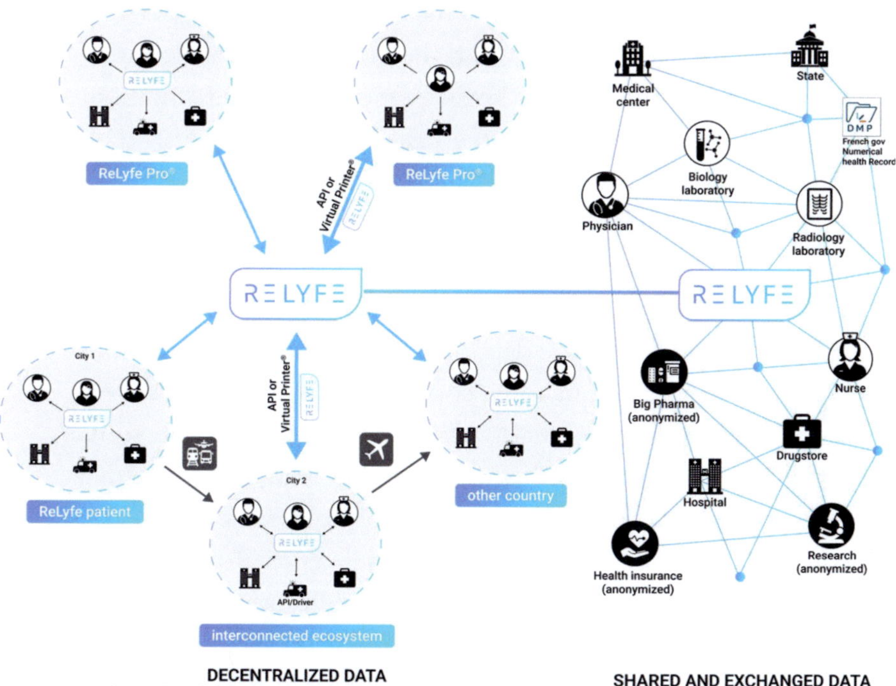

Figure 1: Hybrid technology model proposed in the ReLyfe project

1.1 Context, Observations and Situation Report

A. The Computerization of Health Data

The computerization of health is the foundation of a quality healthcare service, since information technologies can improve both patient care and health systems.

Indeed, an effective healthcare service is patient-information-centered.

Moreover, doctors and healthcare professionals need reliable and relevant data to diagnose diseases, prescribe medication and provide their patients with appropriate advice. Likewise, managers rely on quality information to make right decisions.

For example, the management of the necessary hospital personnel, facilities and drug stocks, and the effective management of epidemics relies on the sound management of this information. In many countries with effective health systems, healthcare is founded on a solid health information system. Furthermore, the computerization of health systems ensures adequate management of the data healthcare professionals and establishments need to provide their care effectively. Well-functioning information systems allow data to be communicated and synchronized and actions to be coordinated between the different healthcare professionals. With the abundance of tools available in this digital age, a great many potentially informative electronic data sources are currently being amassed in the health sector. Californian group Kaiser Permanente, for instance, which has over 9 million patients, purportedly has between 26.5 and 44 petabytes of health data.

In countries where the provision of medical care is less efficient, the advent of information technology has served to improve healthcare services. Indeed, the World Health Organization (WHO) has already provided Mongolia with computers to improve the country's healthcare system. Likewise, Africa is making continuous improvements in this area with the advent of the Internet and the use of mobile phones, with a high penetration rate and the boom of social media and networks.

However, the rate at which electronic health records are being generated is currently so high, and the type and complexity of this data so diverse, that it can no longer be processed using mainstream software or conventional data management tools and methods.

B. Big Data, Health Data Structuring and Centralization

Although businesses are the major players in the use and application of big data, the health sector has recently become very active in this area. In many cases, big data applications have contributed to cutting costs, from diagnosis and the prescription of appropriate treatments to health system surveillance and better public health accountability. Now, doctors have traditionally used their experience and judgement to make diagnoses and clinical decisions. However, in this digital age of big data, the decisions healthcare professionals make can be machine-guided. Indeed, patient data and information generated by other healthcare professionals, specifically laboratories and radiology, are transmitted in good time, increasing the data available for making more informed decisions about patients. It is this diverse collection of generated data that constitutes the renowned

"Big Data". In the health sector, this data covers clinical data, doctors' prescriptions and notes, medical imaging, the results of biological examinations and laboratory tests, pharmaceutical records, health insurance reports, administrative reports, patient historical data with their personal and family history, as well as publications on social media platforms like Facebook and Twitter, blogs and other information not directly connected to patients, such as news in health magazines, and relevant publications in medical journals. Just like in the business world, the availability of big data in the health sector provides an opportunity to discover relationships, models and trends in data. Information from these sources can therefore improve healthcare. However, this big data poses several key problems, specifically its scattered nature, its lack of structuring, its centralization in databases and software that are not interconnected, the lack of interoperability and, above all, the compartmentalized way the medical world operates.

C. The Limitations of State Siloed "Dossiers Médicaux Partagés" [Shared Health Records] ("DMP")

According to a study conducted by French market research company Opinion Way, almost 70% of patients would like to be able to make online appointments and access and manage an electronic health record. Almost 85% say they are willing to share their health data online. However, the day-to-day management of health records could be improved because 50% of French people do not bring their complete record to their consultations with a healthcare professional, 39% do not know whether their vaccinations are up to date, and 25% only scan and archive their medical analyses.

In France, the government has recently implemented a strategy to transform the health system by speeding up the digital transition. According to the Ministry of Health, these reforms aim to "improve the quality of healthcare for patients and improve day-to-day practice for professionals thanks to the organizational changes they will permit".

Nonetheless, the experience of implementing a shared health record in France has so far been extremely complex. Launched in 2004 by former Minister of Health Philippe Douste-Blazy, this shared medical record has taken 18 years to get under way, and current figures indicate that although around 6 million records have been opened (mainly by pharmacists, paid to do so) only 1% contain clinical and health data. The social security system recently took over the management of this shared medical record after repeated failures by the "Agence des Systèmes Informatiques Partagés en Santé" [Shared Health Information Systems Agency] ("ASIP-Santé") governed by the Ministry of Health. The health insurance system now automatically provides each opened file with two years of reimbursement data history. Moreover, several years ago the "Dossier Pharmaceutique" [Pharmaceutical Record] ("DP") created by the "Ordre National des Pharmaciens" [National Pharmacists Association] succeeded in connecting patients' pharmaceutical pathway. This pharmaceutical record can be opened free of charge in pharmacies with the patient's oral consent. It does not contain clinical information and it is stored for four months. At present, however, the shared health record and pharmaceutical record are not connected, creating discontinuity in the patient care pathway and adding a further barrier to the sharing of health data which remains compartmentalized in each information system.

Actually, there are three major limitations to the effective functioning of shared health records:

1) The absence of a unified digital health identifier.
2) The reluctance of healthcare professionals to fill in a state health record.
3) The market presence of a host of different software publishers for each profession which do not conform to a unique data structuring and interoperability framework.

The patient does not ultimately have efficient and continuous digital access to their medical and paramedical data.

Worldwide, only Australia, Estonia, Israel and a few north European countries have successfully nationalized a basic shared health record, even though we are in an age where technology allows data to be shared, secured, structured and analyzed in most other fields. The medical world is far behind.

MATERIALS AND METHODS

We first carried out a general systematic review and comparison of our own work with the scientific literature using the following key words (via the MeSH and BnF thesauri):

Patient Generated Health Data, Personal Health Records, Telemedicine, Big Data, Artificial Intelligence, Renal Cell Carcinoma, Infrared Spectroscopy, Machine Learning, Data Mining, Deep Learning, Optical Character Recognition, Predictive Medicine.

Initial research work was then carried out since 2015 in the form of a case-control, multi-center pilot study to evaluate the prognostic value of infrared vibrational microscopy in renal carcinoma, by developing a metastatic risk prediction algorithm. This study was conducted on a retrospective cohort of 100 patients with clear cell renal cell carcinoma who had undergone radical nephrectomy with R0 negative surgical margins (no tumor at the margin, no cancer cells seen microscopically at the primary tumor site), divided into two groups: M1 metastatic patients and M0 non-metastatic patients, after five years of follow-up and with matching of the Fuhrman histoprognostic nuclear grade and tumor stage.

The two groups were comparable in terms of their clinical, biological, and histological characteristics. A big data model with 4 million spectral data sets was generated.
The processing and machine learning phase began with k-Means (KM) unsupervised mathematical classification, followed by a comparative statistical analysis of the two groups.

Lastly, considering the initial observations, the obstacles encountered and the results of the first study, a second application work was instigated in 2016 as part of a project to develop a health card called ReLyfe benefiting from a new hybrid technology architecture for sharing and structuring health information.

Four years (2016–2019) were then dedicated to the initial creation of this model, which required the recruitment of a team of specialized engineers within a French corporate structure called ReLyfe Group, which was funded by various research programs of French Public Investment Bank Bpifrance, healthcare professionals, business angels and other private investors.

So, this whole first step took a total of five years of R&D (2015–2019) and led to a successful POC, and then two years (2020-2021) to validating and applying this solution in real-life with a business model.

PART TWO

REVIEW OF THE LITERATURE ON HEALTH BIG DATA

THE CUTTING EDGE OF
HEALTH BIG DATA

Big Data looks very promising for the health sector, bringing with it advantages for analyzing large volumes of a variety of data to obtain accurate information that will allow healthcare professionals and administrators to make better decisions.

Big Data Analytics in healthcare can reveal associations, patterns and trends that enable healthcare providers and stakeholders to better control costs, improve diagnosis and find and use better targeted therapies for diseases.

It can be used for the surveillance and prevention of epidemics and can lead to an overall improvement in patient care, especially in regions like Africa and Middle East.

In 2012, the United States Government invested around 200 million dollars in a big data initiative, with the development of open-access (Open Data) health data analytics to improve medical research and promote scientific innovation (White House, 2012).

As a result, many health-related organizations have begun requesting funding for the use and exploitation of these mega volumes of accessible health information.

Big Data is generally characterized by the 4 Vs (Figure 2): Volume (large quantity of data or big data), Velocity (speed of data change), Variability (different sources of data) and Veracity (degree of reliability of the information).

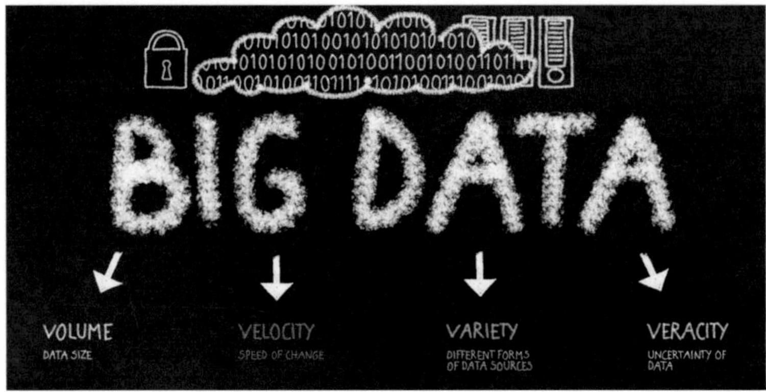

Figure 2: The criteria of big data: 4 Vs

Although the application of healthcare big data is still in its infancy in Africa for example compared with its application in the developed world, the scientific literature shows that the analysis of large volumes of health data is also emerging in several developing countries, since it can be a key weapon for improving access to healthcare and eradicating many of the diseases prevailing in the African continent.

So, if we take the example of Africa, although many regions do not have the necessary infrastructures or facilities to provide quality healthcare, the growing use of social networks (Facebook, Twitter, WhatsApp, WeChat, etc.), mobile devices and the Internet are generating a significant amount of data that can be used for disease surveillance.

In fact, a 2010 United Nations (UN) report shows that Africa has made a giant leap with a high telecommunications penetration rate directly to mobile phones bypassing landlines, thus facilitating the collection of a large volume of data on people's behavior, particularly in relation to disease surveillance.

Digital epidemiology is an emerging field in the public health sector which deals with the way in which big data can be used to detect, understand and identify public health challenges.

With the growing use of social networks and mobile phones, efforts to examine the way big data from these social media and smartphones can be used to simply monitor, prevent, detect and treat diseases can now be stepped up.

By way of example, when around 553 million tweets in the United States were collected online and sorted using key words linked to the Human Immunodeficiency Virus (HIV), analysis results show that there was a high positive correlation between the tweets related to HIV and the HIV cases reported in certain regions of the United States. This demonstrates the value of this social network data as a disease evaluation and prevention tool. Although contagious diseases represent a tremendous burden to the African health sector, big data analytics provides a unique opportunity to monitor the transmission risk of these diseases. During the Ebola crisis, mobile phones were one of the most useful tools.

Indeed, smartphones are widely available in many African countries, including the regions affected by the Ebola virus. Scientists therefore exploited the very rich data source provided by mobile phone companies to visualize the movements of Ebola patients and predict how the virus could spread.

A telecommunications provider in an affected West African country, for example, provided Swiss Non-Governmental Organization (NGO) flow minder with the anonymized voice calls and SMS of around 150,000 mobile phones. Data that was ultimately used to produce detailed epidemiological maps illustrating the movements of patients with the Ebola virus. The authorities then used this information to determine the best locations to set up treatment centers and deployed measures to limit movements to control the disease's spread.

Then there is the important notion of Business Intelligence (BI) to address. A tool, a technology, a process, a methodology and an architecture used to collect, store and analyze data to provide more detailed information to aid strategic decision-making.

It has been proven that BI has the capacity to make collected data like health records operational to make an evidence-based medical practice possible, thus improving healthcare provision. Due to our society's dynamics in terms of legislative and regulatory changes and the quantity of data generated, healthcare organizations can use BI solutions to exploit data for effective decision-making, thereby improving patient services, reducing administrative costs and optimizing patient management. Healthcare providers and professionals now manage the health service as if it were a business, making BI of significant interest to this sector.

As an architecture, BI provides a framework showing the processes that connect the internal and external stakeholders within the healthcare environment. The sector's decision-makers therefore need to have knowledge of these processes to understand the usefulness of this innovation. Now, this is a field that is not generally short of data. The challenge therefore consists in transforming this enormous quantity of data into useful information and exploitable knowledge. Hence why BI is relevant to the field of health.

The Obama Affordable Care Act focuses on the quality of the health service rather than the number of patients treated, and when this Act came into force, healthcare providers across America raised their concerns. However, thanks to business intelligence software, these healthcare providers were able to predict the financial and operational costs of this Act and therefore determine how to maintain and even improve their efficiency.

The BI global market in the health sector is estimated at 3.596 billion dollars and could be as high as 4.739 billion dollars. The main factors responsible for this growth are the emergence of health big data, improved healthcare provision and patient satisfaction. The United States dominate the strategic intelligence market in the health sector, followed by the Asian countries: China, India, Singapore and Malaysia which have quickly adopted BI in the health sector. The adoption of health BI is also now emerging in African countries and looks set to flourish with the population's growing use of mobile technologies, social media platforms, the growing adoption of cloud computing and the increasing use of electronic health data within the medical community.

Although the application of big data in Africa is still in its infancy, recent reports have shown that digital surveillance is being used to effectively monitor epidemics.

Despite the ethical issues associated with the use of big data in Africa, the risk of an epidemic spreading can sometimes become a national, or indeed, an international crisis. When measures must be taken to save lives, governments must make political decisions to stop such situations at all costs. Hence why the application of big data was recently deployed in the health sector to eradicate these epidemics. The use of electronic surveillance to detect infectious disease epidemics is a giant leap made recently by health administrators in Africa who have paved the way for the use of big data. Early detection and surveillance are essential to the prevention of infectious diseases.

One example would be HealthMap, a form of digital surveillance used successfully in Africa and across the world. It is an open-source automated electronic information system used to present data on disease epidemics according to geography, time and infectious disease carriers.

Health organizations like WHO rely on systems like HealthMap to detect epidemics. For example, the dreaded Ebola epidemic in West Africa was made known to the whole world on March 14, 2014, after HealthMap retrieved the report of a fatal fever in Guinea from a French information website. Based on this report, Sierra Leone, which shares its border with Guinea, officially declared that the Ebola virus had spread to Sierra Leone on March 23. WHO then declared that the Ebola virus was a serious public health epidemic on August 8, 2014. This surveillance has also helped detect new cases of polio in war-torn north-west Nigeria.

HealthMap's strength as a disease location detection tool lies in its capacity to pool immense, diversified, and unstructured resources.

PART THREE

PREDICTING RISK IN KIDNEY CANCER WITH MACHINE LEARNING

CASE STUDY NO.1: PREDICTING METASTASES IN RENAL CARCINOMA BY DEVELOPING A BIG DATA MODEL

1.2   Introduction

A.   Epidemiology

In France, renal carcinoma (Figure 3) is the sixth most common cancer in men and the third most common urological cancer, responsible for almost 4,000 deaths in France according to the "Institut National du Cancer" [National Cancer Institute] ("*InCa*" *2012*).

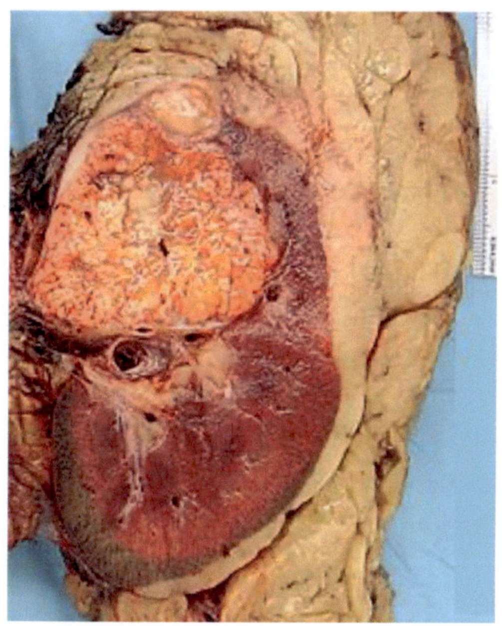

Figure 3: Renal carcinoma tumor piece

B. 2009 TNM Classification

The TNM classification (Table I) is an international system for classifying cancers according to their anatomical extent. Several revisions have been published, the latest used here is the seventh edition in 2009. The letter T stands for the original tumor, the letter N indicates whether or not the tumor has spread to the neighboring lymph nodes, and the letter M refers to the absence or presence of distant metastases.

Table I: 2009 TNM Classification

	TX	Primary tumor cannot be assessed
	T0	No evidence of primary tumor
	T1	Tumor ≤7 cm in greatest dimension, limited to the kidney
		T1a – Tumor ≤4 cm in greatest dimension, limited to the kidney
		T1b – Tumor >4 cm but ≤7 cm in greatest dimension, limited to the kidney
T	T2	Tumor >7 cm in greatest dimension, limited to the kidney
		T2a – Tumor >7 cm but ≤10 cm in greatest dimension, limited to the kidney T2b – Tumor >10 cm, limited to the kidney
	T3	Tumor extends into major veins or perinephric tissues but not into the ipsilateral adrenal gland and not beyond the Gerota fascia

		T3a – Tumor grossly extends into the renal vein or its segmental (muscle-containing) branches, or tumor invades perirenal and/or renal sinus fat but not beyond the Gerota fascia T3b – Tumor grossly extends into the vena cava below the diaphragm T3c – Tumor grossly extends into the vena cava above the diaphragm or invades the wall of the vena cava
	T4	Tumor invades beyond the Gerota fascia (including contiguous extension into the ipsilateral adrenal gland)
N		NX Regional lymph nodes cannot be assessed
		N0 No regional lymph node metastasis
		N1 Metastasis in regional lymph node(s)
		N2 Metastasis in more than 1 regional lymph node
M		MX Distant metastasis cannot be assessed
		M0 No distant metastasis
		M1 Distant metastasis

C. Anatomical Pathology

Histological types of renal tumors:

Clear cell renal cell carcinoma represents 75% of all anatomopathological types of renal carcinoma.

Figure 4 shows the progeny and histo-anatomical origin of the different anatomopathological types of renal carcinoma.

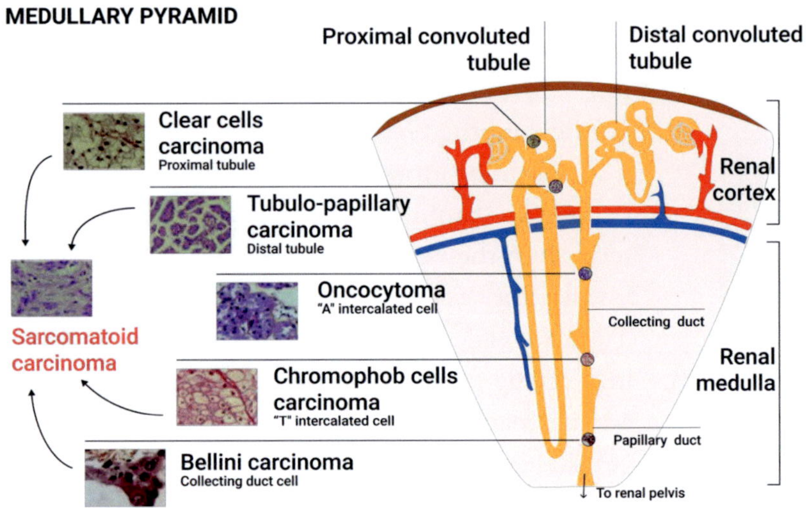

Figure 4: Progeny and anatomopathological origins of renal carcinoma

Figure 5 presents examples of histological sections of the main anatomopathological types of renal carcinoma:

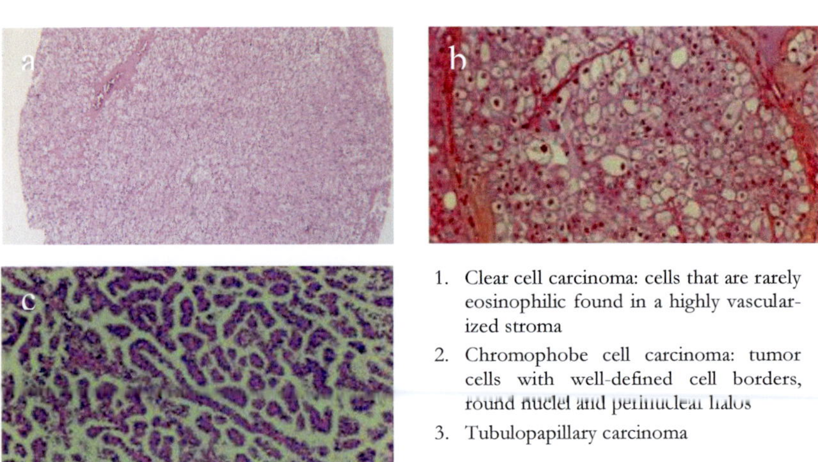

1. Clear cell carcinoma: cells that are rarely eosinophilic found in a highly vascularized stroma
2. Chromophobe cell carcinoma: tumor cells with well-defined cell borders, round nuclei and perinuclear halos
3. Tubulopapillary carcinoma

Figure 5: Histological sections of the main anatomopathological types

Table II compares the characteristics of six types of renal cell tumors:

Table II: Main characteristics of the six anatomopathological types of renal cell tumors

	Frequency	Sex ratio	Origin	Precursor	Bilaterality	Chromosonic abnormality
Clear cell carcinoma	75%	2H/1F	Proximal bypass tube	no		-3p VHL
Tubulo papillary tumor	10%	8H1F	Distal bypass tube	Yes papillary adenoma	yes	+7, +17, -Y +16, +12, +20
Chromophobic cell carcinoma	5%	F>H	Collector tube (Cortical)		no	-1, -2, -13 -3
Oncocytoma	5%	F>H	Collector tube (Cortical)		yes	-1, -14, -19 mitochondrial DNA defects
Bellini's carcinoma	1%	H>F	Collector tube (Extra-pyra-midic)			-1, -6, -14
Carcomatoid carcinoma	1%		bypass tube or collector tube			-8, -9, -14

D. Treatment

The standard treatment is partial or radical nephrectomy depending on the size of the tumor T and the technical feasibility. For the metastatic forms, the treatment strategy chosen, and the role of nephrectomy are currently guided by a prognostic assessment based on clinical and biological criteria. However, these criteria only allow an imprecise evaluation of the prognosis (Table III).

Table III: Summary of the main prognostic systems for renal carcinoma

| | Localized kidney cancer models | | | Metastatic kidney cancer models | |
	UISS	SSICN	Karakiewicz's nomogram	MSKCC model (2002)	Heng model
TNM stage	X	X	X		
ECOG or Kamofsky	X			X	X
Symptoms related to cancer			X		
Fuhrman grade	X	X	X		
Tumor necrosis		X			
Tumor size		X	X		
Time from diagnosis to treatment				X	X
LDH				X	
Corrected calcium				X	X
Hemoglobin				X	X
Neutrophils					X
Platelets					X
Prognostic accuracy	0.81	0.82	0.86	ND	0.73

In the last few years, tyrosine kinase inhibitors have emerged as a treatment for the metastatic forms. This inhibitor blocks the activity of tyrosine kinase, an enzyme involved in the cell signaling process. Tyrosine kinase plays a role in cell communication, development, division, and growth. Tyrosine kinase inhibitors are therefore a type of targeted therapy by inhibiting the growth factor and angiogenesis. Standard chemotherapy cannot be used to treat renal carcinoma. Anti-angiogenic targeted therapies have doubled the progression-free survival time from five to ten months, although median survival remains low at eight months. However, the cost of these new therapies is very high. Moreover, the treatment response is uncertain, and several lines of treatment remain necessary.

E. Prognosis

The prognosis is closely linked to the tumor's aggressiveness and the onset of secondary distant metastatic lesions. In fact, the five-year survival rate decreases from 70% for the M0 non-metastatic forms to 10% for the M1 metastatic forms. Clinicians currently have access to very little accurate and objective information to evaluate this prognosis, and for the moment the Fuhrman grade remains at the forefront. It is an independent prognosis factor but is subject to inter-individual anatomopathological interpretation variability which impairs its reproducibility and relevance. The Fuhrman grade is based on the nuclear atypia of the most atypical contingent of cells, and cell type and tumor architecture are not considered. This grade integrates 4 parameters: the size of the nuclei (from 10 to 20 microns), the contours of the nuclei (regular, irregular), the presence of nucleoli at different magnifications (x400, x100) and the presence of bizarre cells (immediately classes the tumor in the highest grade = Fuhrman 4).

The system has 4 grades of increasing severity (Figure 6).
Two different anatomical pathologists have a 5% risk of giving two different interpretations.

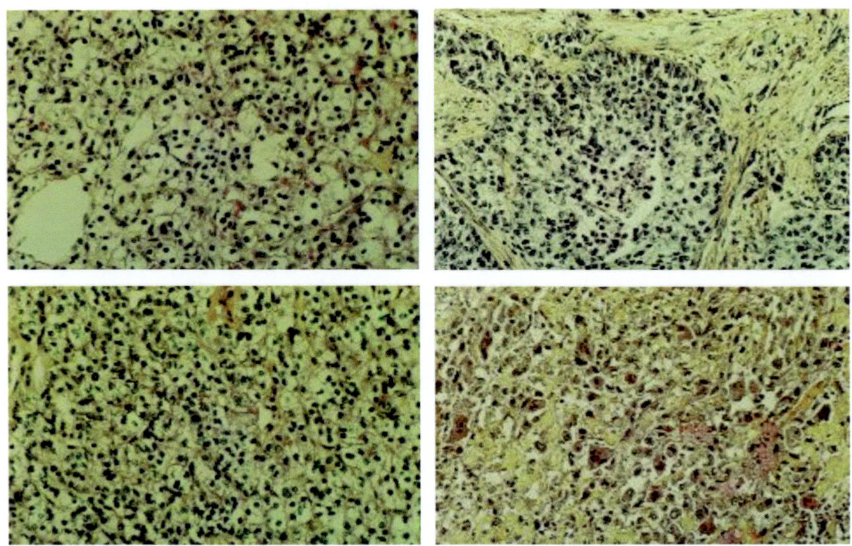

Figure 6: The 4 grades of Fuhrman's anatomopathological grading system

Now in practice, from a prognostic perspective, we can separate low-grade renal cell cancers (1 and 2) which have a five-year survival rate of over 70%, and high-grade cancers (3 and 4) which have a five-year survival rate of less than 50%.

The onset of metastases increases with the grade:
- Grade 1 (Figure 6, top left): 2%
    The nuclei are small and regular, the nucleoli are not visible.
- Grade 2 (Figure 6, top right): 9%
    The nuclei are larger and irregular, the nucleoli will be visible at a higher magnification (x400).
- Grade 3 (Figure 6, bottom right): 17%

The nuclei are large and prominent and very irregular, the nucleoli will be visible at a lower magnification (x100).

- Grade 4 (Figure 6, bottom right): 30%

The cells are giant, nuclei appear bizarre and multilobate.

The identification of new more reliable and more objective prognostic markers would allow better management of renal carcinoma.

1.3   Infrared Vibrational Microscopy

A.   New Tissue Characterization Optical Technology

The principle of infrared microscopy is based on the absorption of infrared radiation by the tissue's molecular components. Combined with a mapping system, this technique is used to record multidimensional spectral images with a resolution of a few micrometers. Each pixel of the image is composed of a specific infrared spectrum of the biomolecular and structural composition of the tissue at this site.

This technique relies on the possibility of revealing biochemical and molecular changes that occur during physio pathological processes like carcinogenesis. It is a non-destructive, label-free technique.

The molecular information within tissues can be detected by vibrational spectroscopy, even before the tissue's morphology is affected, and therefore at a stage that is undetectable in conventional pathology. Multivariate infrared imaging data processing statistical methods have now been developed for this purpose, paving the way for the concept of Spectral Histo-Pathology (SHP).

Certain developed algorithms authorize the direct analysis of paraffin-embedded samples, by performing digital deparaffinization of the infrared spectra of tissues. The SHP approach therefore seems complementary to conventional histology, allowing for automated tissue characterization that is completely independent of the operator or the anatomical pathologist's evaluation.

This approach can also be used to associate infrared spectral signatures with different tissue components. The analysis of the vibration bands characteristic of these signatures can provide access to the molecular components (collagen, nucleic acids, sugars, etc.) of the tissues.

B. Biophysical Aspects

There are two types of vibrational microscopies:
- Raman Scattering
- Infrared Absorption

Their use as new and complementary tissue characterization tools for application in a clinical setting is steadily on the rise.
The technique we used in this work is infrared absorption vibrational microscopy based on the light-matter interaction in the infrared range. The information obtained is recorded in the form of spectra representing the absorption according to the number of molecular vibration waves.
The statistical processing of this spectral information can then be used to probe the composition and/or structure of large classes of biomolecules present in the sample, in particular proteins, carbohydrates, and nucleic acids.
This technique is based on the measurement of the specific vibrational frequencies of molecules when probed by excitation radiation. A polyatomic molecule has several degrees of freedom for the chemical bond vibration modes. According to the incident radiation frequency, these bonds will undergo different vibration modes: elongation, angular bending, or out-of-plane bending (Figure 7).

The figure 7 below shows an example of the different vibration waves of the CH2 group.

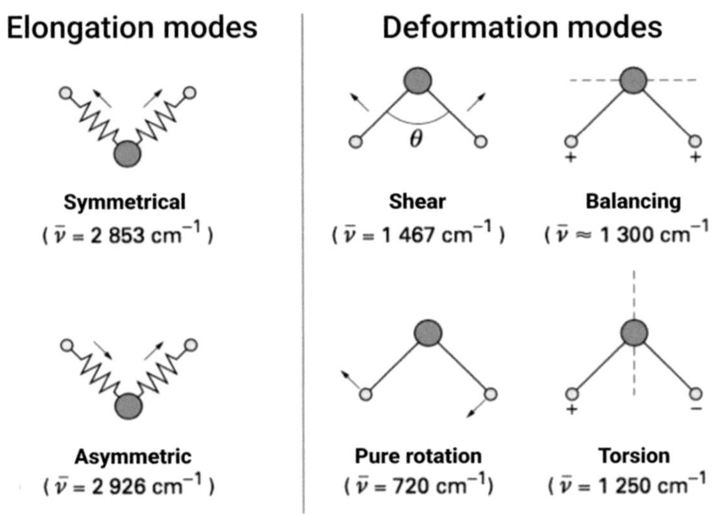

Figure 7: Vibration waves of the CH2 group

Infrared absorption vibrational spectroscopy consists in measuring the energy variations between the incident radiation and the radiation after interaction with the sample. It can then be used to obtain the intensity variations of each of these vibration modes. These variations are represented in the form of a spectrum, which can be considered a digital fingerprint containing the biomolecular information specific to the sample.

When the energy from the light radiation passing through the sample is equal to the vibrational energy of the atomic bonds of one of its molecules, the radiation is partially absorbed, decreasing its intensity. An infrared spectrum therefore contains absorption A (or transmittance T) values according to the number of waves expressed in cm^{-1}.

The IR radiation domain is comprised of three regions:

- Near-IR: 12,500 – 400 cm^{-1}
- Mid-IR: 4,000 – 400 cm^{-1}
- Far-IR: 400 – 10 cm^{-1}

Mid-IR corresponds to the vibration frequency domain of the bonds of most of the molecules, and therefore represents the region most suited to biomolecular analysis.

The figure below (Figure 8) shows an example of the Mid-IR absorption spectrum of the different structures of a biological sample. Figure 9 shows the attribution of the vibrational modes of the main organic compounds.

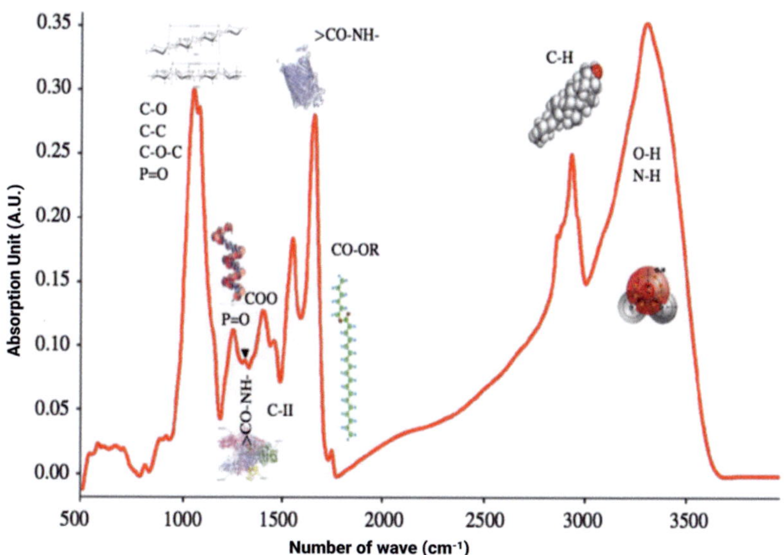

Figure 8: IR absorption spectrum of a biological sample

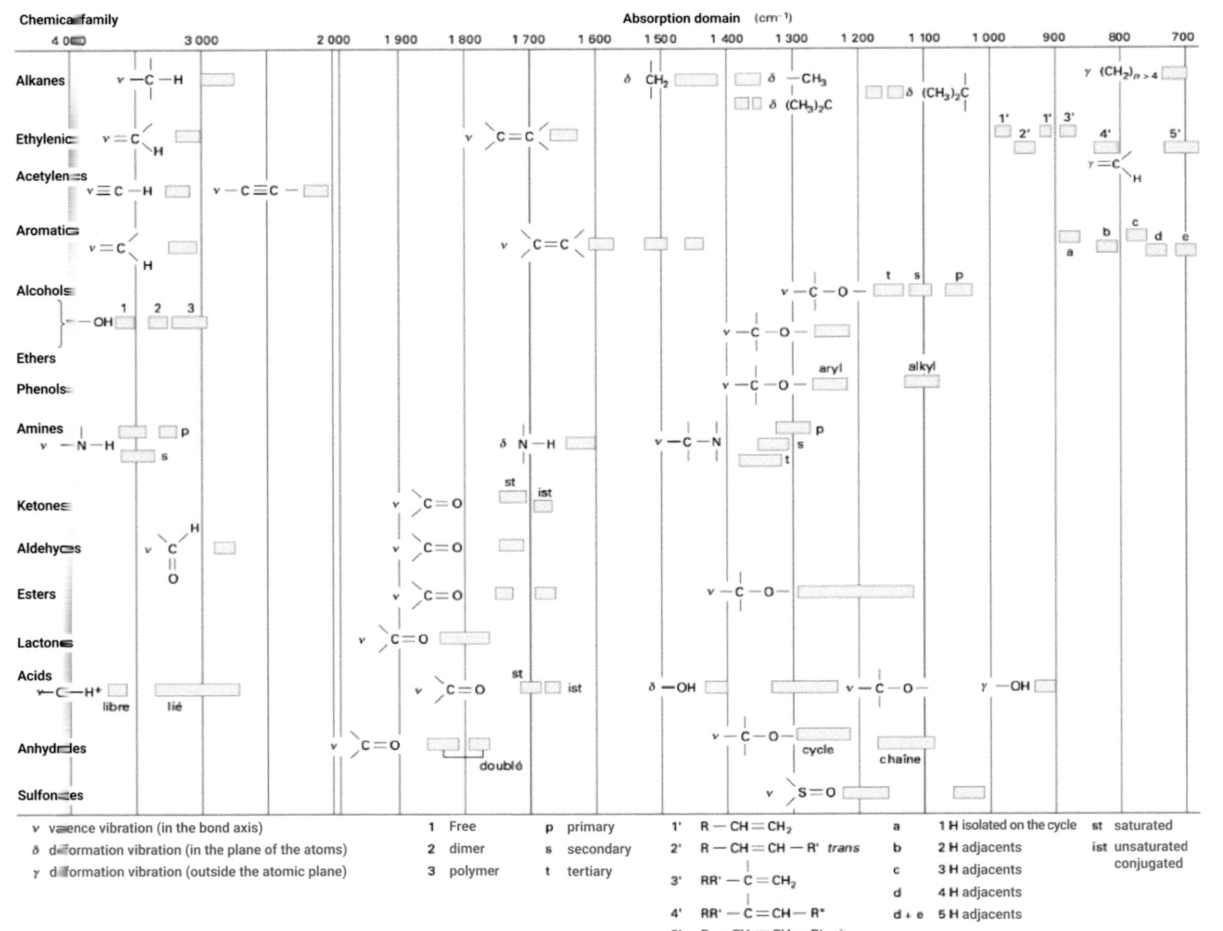

Figure 9: Attribution of the vibrational modes of the main organic compounds

1.4   Study Rationale

In this work we focused on prognosis by studying tumor aggressiveness in renal cell carcinoma. The rationale for this research project is the use of this innovative biophotonic technology: infrared microscopy, to respond to a well-defined clinical question, i.e., the prediction of renal tumor invasiveness by developing a big data model. The optical big data will then be statistically analyzed by machine learning to establish a clustering of tissues according to pre- and post-defined criteria (Figure 10).

Although the proof of concept of the practical potential of this approach has been published, its use in urologic oncology remains limited. Yet, the current scientific literature shows that it has potential valuable applications in urologic oncology for the bladder, kidney and prostate, particularly for in-vitro diagnosis.

Vibrational spectroscopy, which has demonstrated its potential in tumor diagnosis, notably renal, could be a promising tool for the prognostic evaluation of tumors. However, to our knowledge, no study has yet been published on this subject.

SPECTROSCOPY

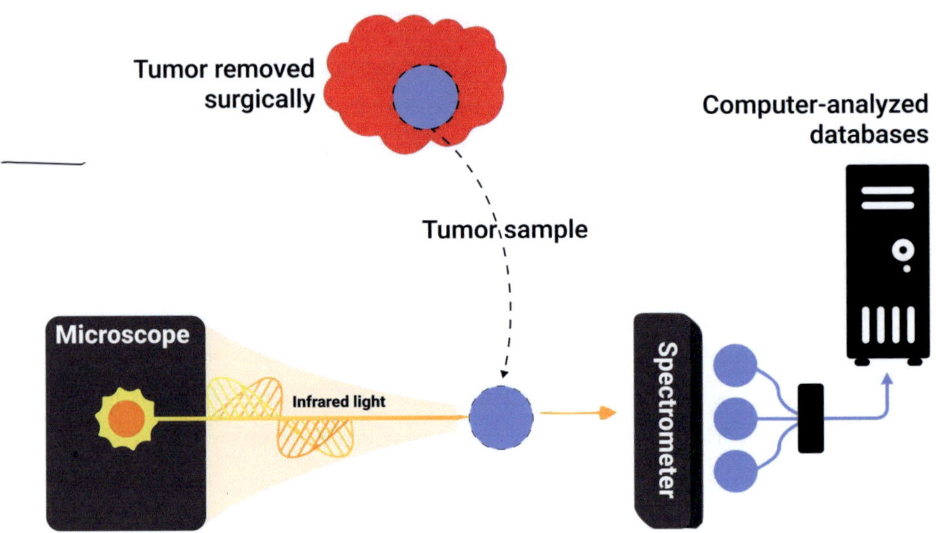

Figure 10: Acquisition of tumor big data by microscopy

1.5   Objective

The primary objective of this project was to establish by infra-red microscopy a characteristic spectral signature that can be used to define a prognostic optical marker for clear cell renal cell carcinoma.

1.6   Materials and Methods

A.   Study Design and Patient Selection

Our study is a case-control, multi-center, prognostic pilot study carried out retrospectively on a cohort of 100 patients having undergone an R0 radical nephrectomy (healthy/clean surgical margins) for clear cell renal cell carcinoma between 2005 and 2010 and monitored for at least five years until 2015, in three centers: Reims University Hospital, Tenon Hospital in Paris, and the Institute for Cancer Control Jean Godinot in Reims where patients are monitored once they transition to metastatic stage.

The first-line treatment these patients receive at these centers is a tyrosine kinase inhibitor.

Two groups of 50 patients were created with matching for two confounding factors: Tumor T size and the Fuhrman nuclear grade (Grade 1, 2, 3 or 4). A first "control" group comprised of patients without M0 recurrent metastasis after at least five years of monitoring. A second "case" group containing M1 metachronous metastatic patients (having progressed during their monitoring) treated with the same tyrosine kinase inhibitor.

Inclusion Criteria:

- Patients with clear cell renal cell carcinoma.
- Patients having had an R0 radical nephrectomy (negative surgical margins).
- M1 metachronous metastatic patients (having progressed to a secondary metastatic state during post-nephrectomy monitoring).
- Patients receiving a tyrosine kinase inhibitor as a first-line anti-angiogenic targeted therapy (they all received Sunitinib: Sutent®).

Exclusion Criteria:

- R1 patients (invaded positive surgical margins).
- M1 synchronous metastatic patients (immediate discovery of the metastasis, at the time of diagnosis).
- Patients with non-clear cell renal cancers.

The flow chart in Figure 11 provides a summary of the study design.

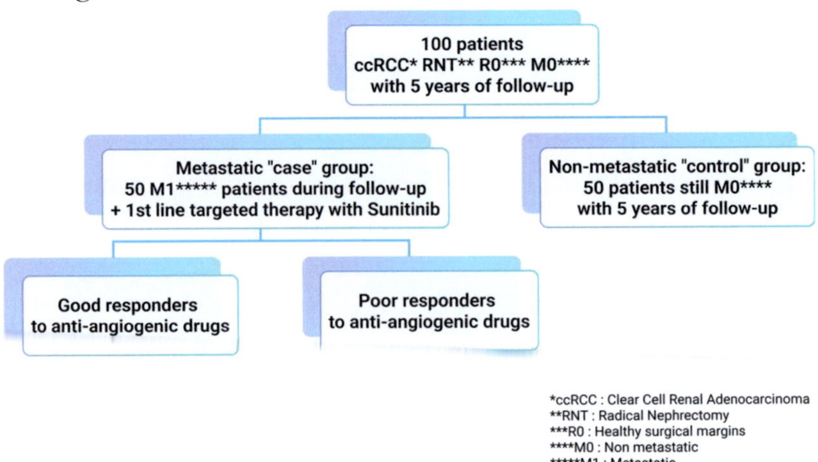

Figure 11: Flow chart summarizing the study design

It should be noted that the patients are matched for tumor T stage and Fuhrman histoprognostic nuclear grade. The data was collected from patients in three centers: Reims University Hospital, Tenon Hospital in Paris and the Institute for Cancer Control Jean Godinot in Reims.

We then investigated three histological zones located on the initial nephrectomy pieces to study the tumor and peritumoral tissue.
- Tumor zone: T.
- Healthy zone located in the peritumoral normal renal parenchyma: H.
- Junction zone between the healthy part and the tumor part (mixed zone): J.

B.   Data Acquisition

Data acquisition is divided into several stages to create Tissue MicroArray (TMA) cores:

a)   Identification of Cores on Biological Samples

Microscopic identification of the blocks of interest on the histological sections stained with Hematoxylin-Eosin-Saffron (HES), then identification of the corresponding areas of interest on each block: 2 Tumor (T) zones, a Healthy zone core (H = renal parenchyma) and a Junction zone core (J = mixed including healthy zone, tumor zone, junction between the two and peritumoral stroma). This phase was carried out at the Reims University Hospital Biopathology Laboratory with blinded double reading including an experienced urologic pathologist.
The cores were then duplicated as a precautionary measure.

b)   **Preparation of the Tissue MicroArrays**

Completion of 13 TMAs on specific Calcium Fluoride (CaF_2) slides suitable for infrared analysis. This phase was carried out with the help of a technician at the INSERM Laboratory U903, Reims Champagne-Ardenne University (URCA).

Spectral Acquisition was performed on these TMAs carried out from tissue samples.

These tissue samples derived from the initial nephrectomies were fixed in Formalin then embedded in Paraffin. A 1-mm diameter needle, computer-guided by the Easy TMA Creator[®] software version 3 (Figure 12) was used to sample a cylindrical tissue core from the source block corresponding to a previously selected zone of interest. Using the same needle and software, this tissue core was then inserted into a target block. The target block could therefore contain up to 80 TMA cores. Two sections were then taken from this block. Two adjacent thin sections are taken: the first section is placed on CaF_2 media (CRYSTRAN, UK) suitable for infrared analyses, the second is stained with HES.

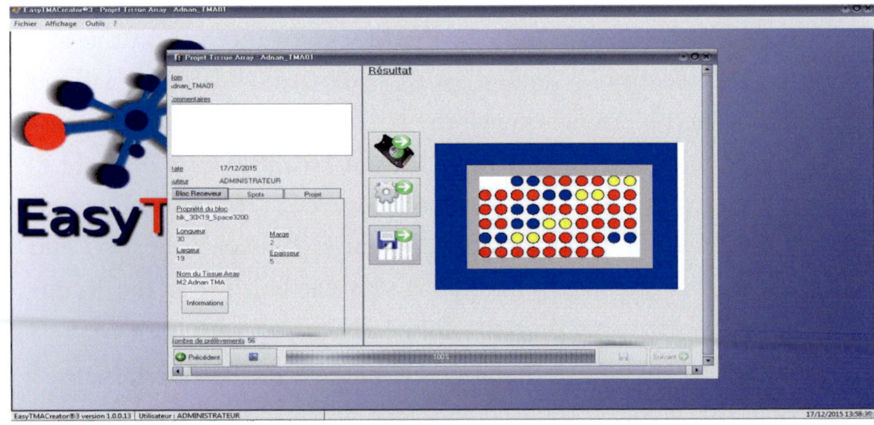

Figure 12: Tissue microarray creation software

TMA is a semi-automatic technique that requires a predefined desired architectural plan. The selected paraffin blocks (donor blocks) are inserted into the device then the identified HES slide is laid on top of the block to digitally define the areas of interest using the software which systematically saves a photo at each identification step (Figure 13).

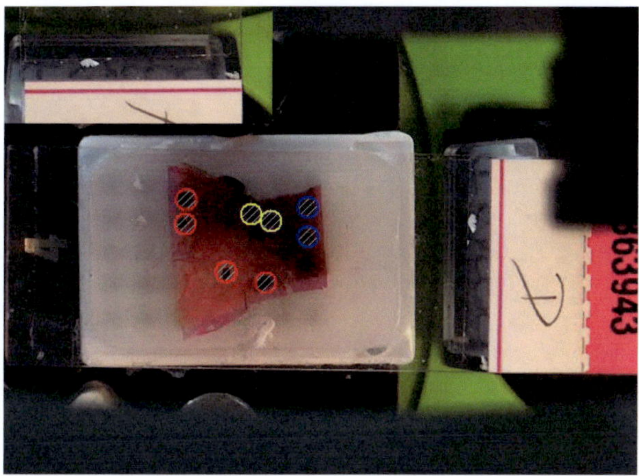

Figure 13: Systematic photo and digital identification of the target areas

A recipient paraffin block is also inserted into the device straight away, this block receives the cores of interest sampled using a needle. The distance between the cores is fixed at 0.5 mm.

C. Sectioning: HES and CaF$_2$

For each TMA recipient block, consecutive 10-μm sections were cut using a microtome. Three were placed on standard glass slides for HES staining and other potential analyses, and one section was placed on a CaF$_2$ media suitable for infrared spectral imaging analysis.

The CaF_2 section, which is essential to our optical acquisitions, is positioned on the specific CaF_2 media without the use of a fixing agent using a drop of distilled water. This media is then placed on a hot plate until the water is fully evaporated and paraffin liquefaction occurs. The CaF_2 media is used because it does not absorb infrared radiation and therefore allows measurements to be taken in transmission mode for analysis of thin tissue samples. It is important to point out that for the remainder of the spectroscopic analyses, this section on CaF_2 was not chemically deparaffinized or stained.

The HES-stained sections made it possible to identify the histological structures.

This information is crucial to the interpretation of spectral data. A color code was created to identify the cores (Figure 14).

-   Blue = H: Healthy zone of the peritumoral normal renal parenchyma.
-   Red = T: Intra-Tumor zone.
-   Yellow = J: Marginal Junction or transition zone between H and T (mixed).

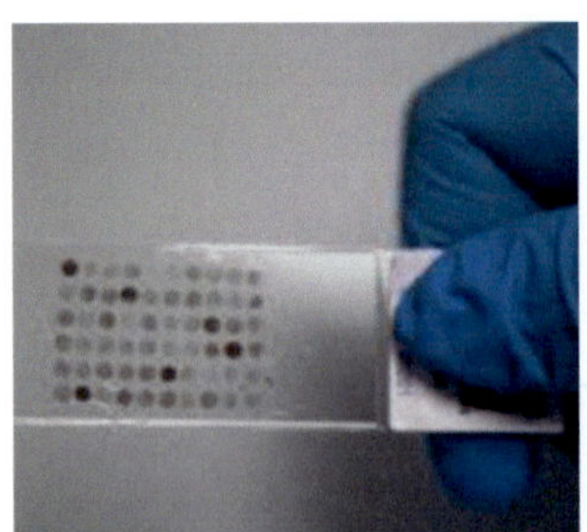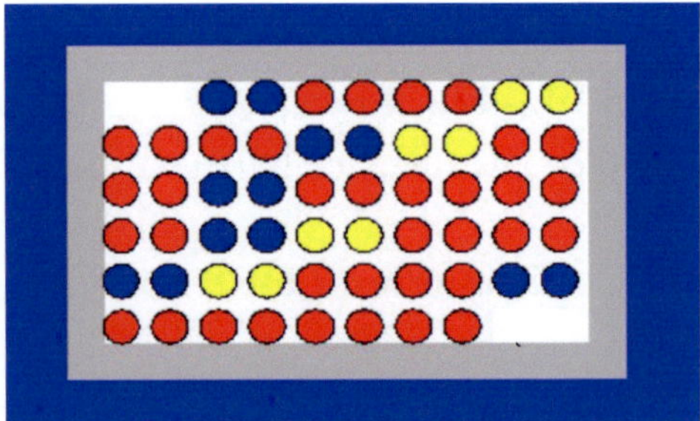

Figure 14: Color code for the identification of cores

D. Infrared Micro-Imaging Analysis

a) Optical Acquisition

The acquisition was performed at the "Biophotonique et Technologies pour la Santé" [Biophotonics and Technologies for Health] Laboratory, Mixed Research Unit 7369 "MEDyC" [Extracellular Matrix and Cellular Dynamics] at the Reims Faculty of Medicine. The equipment used is the Spotlight FT-IR 2. The software used is called Spectrum Image.

Each core generated a spectral image stored in a file. Depending on the spatial resolution, each image contains between 3,000 and 5,000 spectra when the resolution is 25 µm, and between 20,000 and 30,000 spectra when the resolution is 6.25 µm.

Concerning the acquisition parameters, we acquired images of the junction zones of the first 6 TMAs with a better spatial resolution (6.25 µm), assuming that these zones are mixed and diverse compared with the tumor or healthy zones (T and H) which are relatively uniform. As this analysis is very time-consuming, we performed all the next seven TMAs with a spatial resolution of 25 µm, including for the junction zones.

In fact, one 25-µm core requires an average acquisition time of one hour (between 30 minutes and 1 hour and 30 minutes) compared with an average of 6 hours (between 5 and 7 hours) for one 6.25-µm core.

It should be noted that the cores are circular on the TMA slides, however, the acquisition image of each core (marker) is selected using the Spectrum Image software as a square containing the circular core (Figure 15).

	A	B	C	D	E	F	G	H	I	J
1			1 0001 HB273045A Healthy (5200;0)	1 0002 HB273045A Healthy (7800;0)	1 0003 HB273045C Tumor (10400;0)	1 0004 HB273045C Tumor (13000;0)	1 0005 HB273045C Tumor (15600;0)	1 0006 HB273045C Tumor (18200;0)	1 0007 HB273045C Junction (20800;0)	1 0008 HB273045C Junction (23400;0)
2	1 0009 HB363943D Tumor (0;2600)	1 0010 HB363943D Tumor (2600;2600)	1 0011 HB363943D Tumor (5200;2600)	1 0012 HB363943D Tumor (7800;2600)	1 0013 HB363943D Healthy (10400;2600)	1 0014 HB363943D Healthy (13000;2600)	1 0015 HB363943D Junction (15600;2600)	1 0016 HB363943D Junction (18200;2600)	1 0017 HB274449A Tumor (20800;2600)	1 0018 HB274449A Tumor (23400;2600)
3	1 0019 HB274449A Tumor (0;5200)	1 0020 HB274449A Tumor (2600;5200)	1 0021 HB337471H Healthy (5200;5200)	1 0022 HB337471H Healthy (7800;5200)	1 0023 HB337471F Tumor (10400;5200)	1 0024 HB337471F Tumor (13000;5200)	1 0025 HB337471F Tumor (15600;5200)	1 0026 HB337471F Tumor (18200;5200)	1 0027 HB372225E Tumor (20800;5200)	1 0028 HB372225E Tumor (23400;5200)
4	1 0029 HB372225E Tumor (0;7800)	1 0030 HB372225E Tumor (2600;7800)	1 0031 HB372225E Healthy (5200;7800)	1 0032 HB372225E Healthy (7800;7800)	1 0033 HB372225E Junction (10400;7800)	1 0034 HB372225E Junction (13000;7800)	1 0035 HB354921 Tumor (15600;7800)	1 0036 HB354921 Tumor (18200;7800)	1 0037 HB354921 Tumor (20800;7800)	1 0038 HB354921 Tumor (23400;7800)
5	1 0039 HB354921 Healthy (0;10400)	1 0040 HB354921 Healthy (2600;10400)	1 0041 HB354921 Junction (5200;10400)	1 0042 HB354921 Junction (7800;10400)	1 0043 HB377558C Tumor (10400;10400)	1 0044 HB377558C Tumor (13000;10400)	1 0045 HB377558C Tumor (15600;10400)	1 0046 HB377558C Tumor (18200;10400)	1 0047 HB377558B Healthy (20800;10400)	1 0048 HB377558B Healthy (23400;10400)
6	1 0049 HB352716G Tumor (0;13000)	1 0050 HB352716G Tumor (2600;13000)	1 0051 HB352716G Tumor (5200;13000)	1 0052 HB352716G Tumor (7800;13000)	1 0053 HB368175D Tumor (10400;13000)	1 0054 HB368175D Tumor (13000;13000)	1 0055 HB368175D Tumor (15600;13000)	1 0056 HB368175D Tumor (18200;13000)		

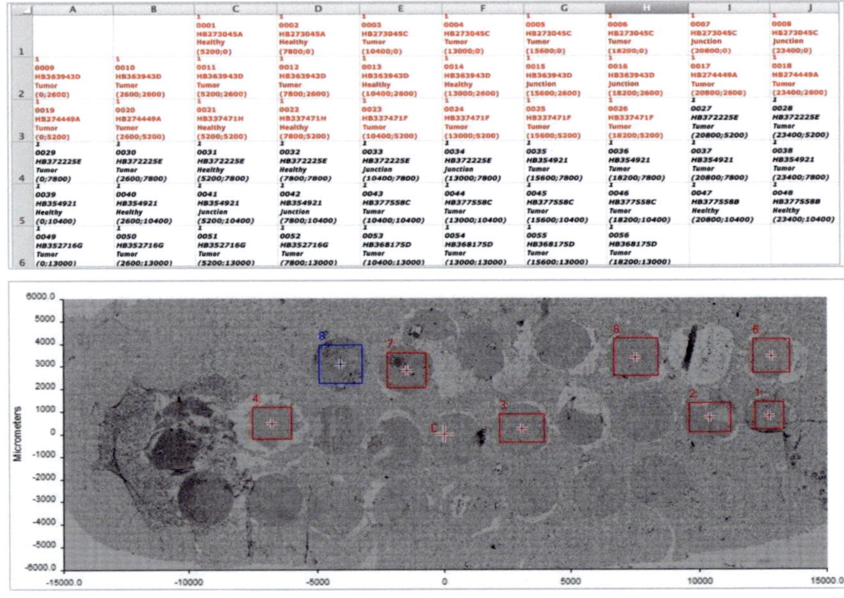

Figure 15: Identification and selection of the tissue target zones for optical acquisition

This acquisition stage requires careful handling of liquid Nitrogen since it must be used for cooling the spectroscopy instrument on a daily basis. This instrument must supply sufficient mean energy of 2,200 Joules for a maximum continuous acquisition of 8 to 10 hours.

Moreover, thirty minutes' calibration time is required when the spectrometer is switched on. It must also be pointed out that there are atmospheric contaminants (water vapor and CO2) inside the acquisition space where the TMA slide is placed, whose spectral contributions will be cancelled out by atmospheric correction (see below – data preprocessing section) before the spectra are analyzed.

b) **Calibration of the Target Dimensions: Format Stage**

Once the instrument has been calibrated and the CaF_2 slide placed in the spectrometer, the TMA dimensions must be entered in the "Format Stage" section so that all of the cores can be scanned to mark the tissue to be targeted for Optical Acquisition (Figure 16).

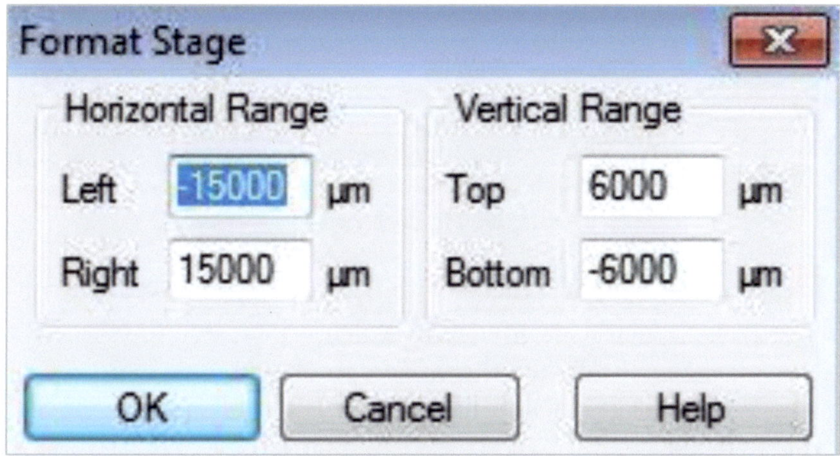

Figure 16: Format Stage

c) **Background Image**

A background image called "Background" (Figure 17), free of any tissue or paraffin, must be acquired for each TMA, on a clean area of the CaF_2 slide.

In transmission mode, this reference spectra called "Background" was therefore recorded prior to each acquisition on a

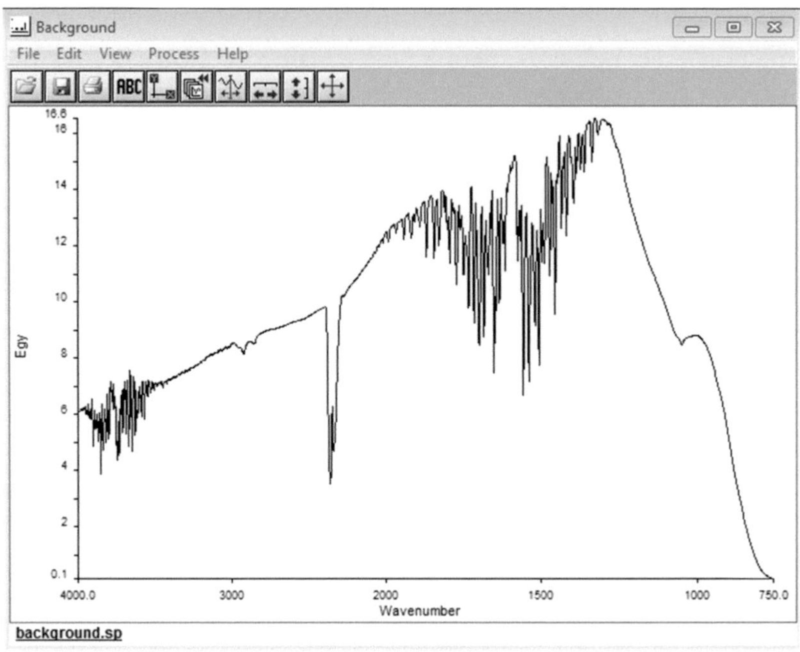

Figure 17: Background

clean area of the CaF$_2$ media with the same optical parameters, except for spectral accumulation which is increased to 60 scans per pixel specifically for this image, to allow better interpretation of the tissue spectra.

This "Background" reference spectra will be automatically subtracted when the tissue spectra containing both the signal from the tissue and the paraffin contribution are generated.

<u>Spectral acquisition parameters:</u>

- Instrument: Perkin Elmer Spotlight 400
- Mean Energy: 2,200 Joules (between 1,800 and 2,400 J)
- Image Mode: Transmittance
- Spatial Resolution: 25 per pixel
- Spectral Resolution: 4 cm^{-1}

-   16 scans per pixel
-   Spectral Range: 4,000 – 750 cm^{-1}

This Spectral Range was selected because it is considered informative for biological samples. Indeed, it comprises a region (from 900 to 1,800 cm^{-1}) which contains the specific spectral bands of the tissue's main biomolecular classes (Figure 18).

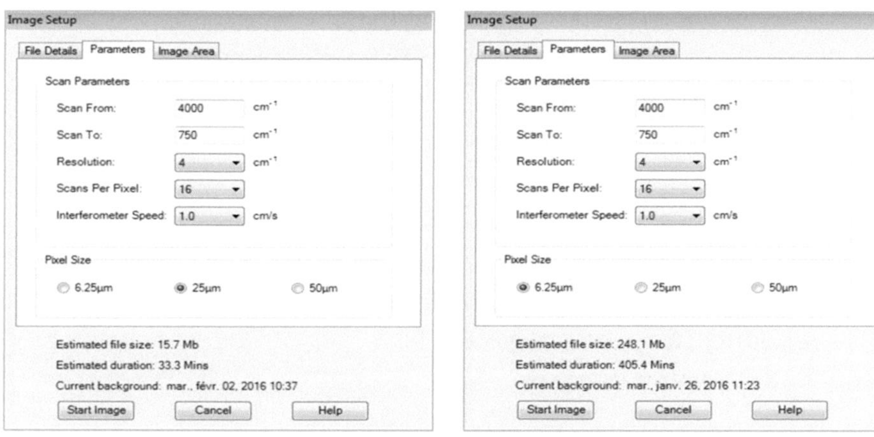

Figure 18: Spectral acquisition parameters

E. Biophysical Aspects of the Instrumentation Used

The infrared spectral images are recorded by a Spotlight micro-imager connected to a Spectrum One (Perkin Elmer) infrared spectrometer.

This system uses a polychromatic light source which is focused with a Cassegrain objective. The micro-imager part has a liquid Nitrogen-cooled detector. It has an inbuilt purging system to minimize the contribution of water vapor and CO2.

To acquire an infrared spectral image, the light source passes through the different points of the sample with two-dimensional scanning. Each image is recorded with a pixel size of 6.25

x 6.25 μm or 25 x 25 μm depending on our chosen spatial resolution, as previously detailed. At each pixel, an infrared absorption spectrum with a spectral range of 4,000 – 750 cm-1 was recorded.

Each spectrum has a spectral resolution of 4 cm-1 and a spectral accumulation of 16 scans per pixel. A spectral image acquired using the "Spectrum Image" software represents a three-dimensional image or data set. The first two dimensions X and Y are the geographic coordinates of each spectrum. The third dimension corresponds to the wave numbers of the Mid-IR spectral range (i.e., each pixel is represented by an IR spectrum).

Figure 19 shows an example of an IR spectral image. This image is equivalent to a data set, where X and Y represent the spatial coordinates of each spectrum, and Λ the different wave numbers of the IR spectral range.

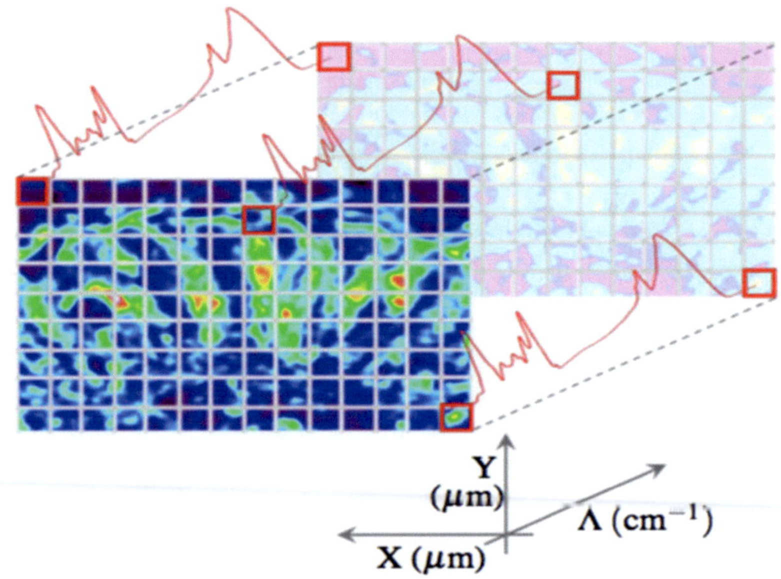

Figure 19: Data set of IR spectral images

Figure 20 shows the IR spectral micro-imager.

The system comprises (A) an imaging system (Spotlight, Perkin Elmer) and (B) a spectrometer (Spectrum One, Perkin Elmer).

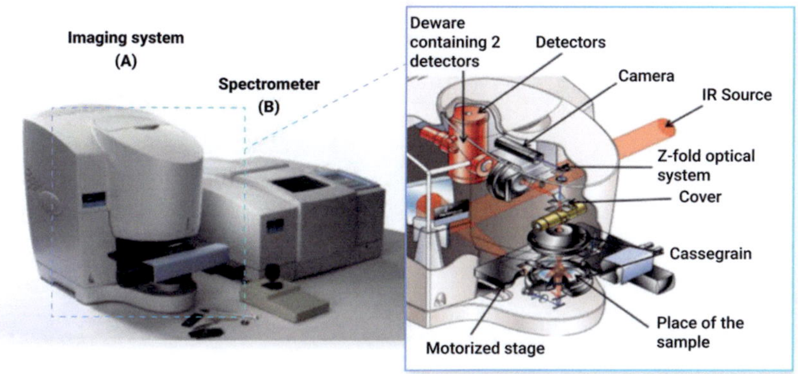

Figure 20: IR spectral micro-imager

a)   **Infrared Absorption**

During this pre-analytical acquisition stage, we observed an infrared absorption difference on these examples of three types of tissue cores (Figure 21): J (Junction), T (Tumor) and H (Healthy).

However, this is only an observation because it cannot be interpreted at this stage and such an absorption difference can, in fact, be due to a variation in section thickness.

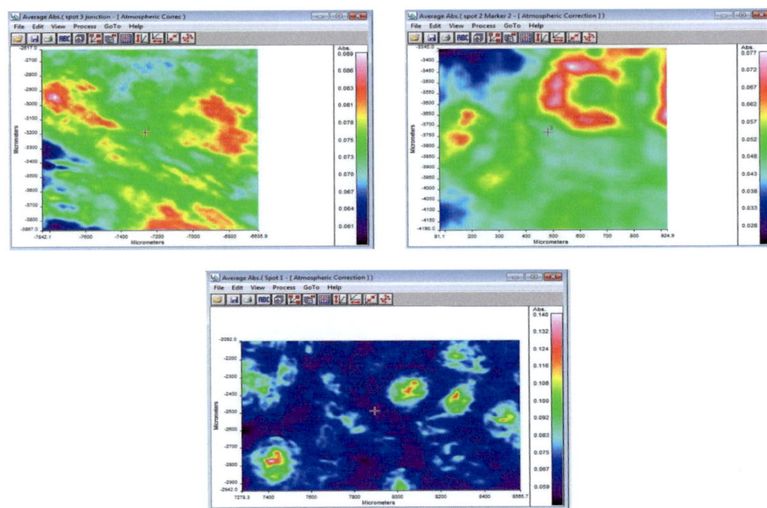

Figure 21: Infrared absorption on three different types of tissue cores

F.   Spectral Data Processing

The spectral images obtained are made up of a very large number of multidimensional spectra. The biological information of interest, often very precise, must be extracted by specific chemometric processing which includes the following main stages:

- <u>Preprocessing</u> of the spectra to eliminate interference while retaining the biomolecular spectral information.

- <u>Unsupervised Classification</u> (or Clustering), to explore the structure of the spectral data by dividing it into homogeneous groups (stage performed here).

<u>Supervised Classification</u> (or Deep Learning Predictive Algorithms - to be created), used to develop a model capable of learning to automatically predict the status of a spectra (stage to be envisaged later as part of a continuation of this work).

The different digital processing stages of the spectral images were performed using programs written in MATLAB® language, which is the software used in this work, with the help of a biomathematician and a biocomputer scientist.
This digital processing is multivariate.

a)   **Preprocessing Stage**

1. Atmospheric Correction

For each spectral image, the contributions of atmospheric contaminants (water vapor and CO_2) are corrected by the "Spectrum Image" software (Figure 22).

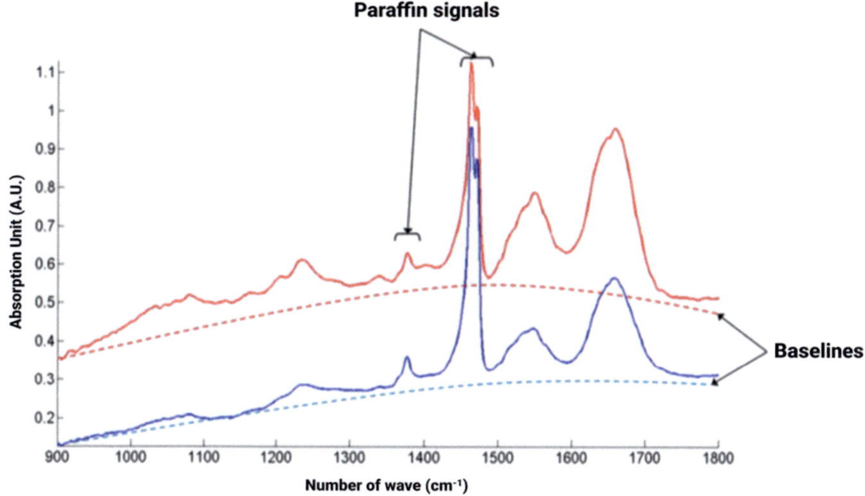

Figure 22: Examples of infrared spectra on a Paraffin-embedded tissue section

2. Extended Multiplicative Signal Correction (EMSC) Protocol

The spectra acquired from the Paraffin-embedded tissue sections are polluted by light scattering caused by the sample and the signal from the Paraffin. These effects produce intense spectral bands and a scattered baseline which differ from one spectrum to the next.

These two effects were simultaneously corrected for our work by EMSC according to an established, validated, and published Protocol. This consists of digital deparaffinization (Figure 23) by mathematical neutralization of the Paraffin contributions because the variability of the signals from the Paraffin affects how the tissue information can be exploited. To do this, we performed an additional acquisition of a 10 x 10 mm^2 square on Paraffin peripheral to the tissue on each TMA slide.

This processing therefore neutralizes the variabilities of the baseline and the pure signal of the paraffin, the latter being detected within the spectral image and eliminated during the digital analyses.

The usual spectral analysis stages were then carried out for the data's interpretation, i.e., first of all, KM Unsupervised Classification.

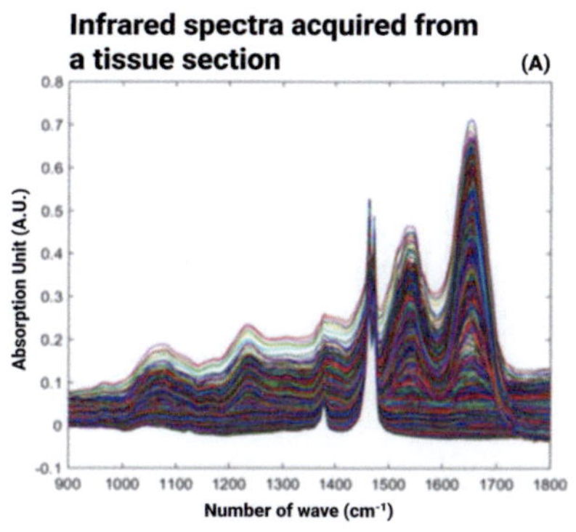
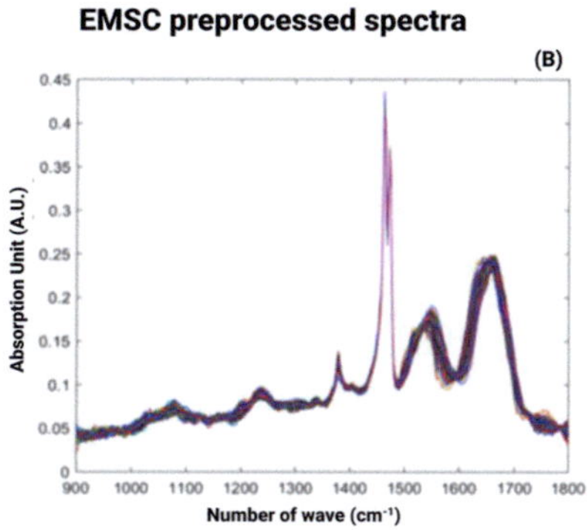

Figure 23: Result of digital deparaffinization after EMSC preprocessing

b)   KM Unsupervised Classification

Following EMSC correction, the KM unsupervised classification method is applied to the spectra to identify the histological structures present in the analyzed sample. It is a clustering method used to partition a data set comprised of many different spectra of such dimensions into k classes (or clusters) by minimizing intra-cluster variation. This KM can thus be used to estimate a partition comprised of k classes to which the algorithm randomly attributes colors.

We performed a common KM. This algorithm uses what are called validity indexes. A validity index is a mathematical function used to measure the quality of a partition estimated by an unsupervised classification algorithm like KM by calculating the ratio between the distances between the points belonging to the same class and the distances between the points belonging to different classes. Applied to partitions estimated on the same data set, a validity index can be used to find the optimal number of classes.

The validity index used in this work was the PBM (Pakhira-Bandyopadhyay-Maulik).

By HES staining the corresponding section, each spectral color generated by the KM can be specifically attributed to a given histological structure. The KM therefore identifies the spectral signatures of the different tissue structures.

The diagram in Figure 24 summarizes the sequence of protocols and the standard procedure for processing a large volume of multidimensional spectral data.

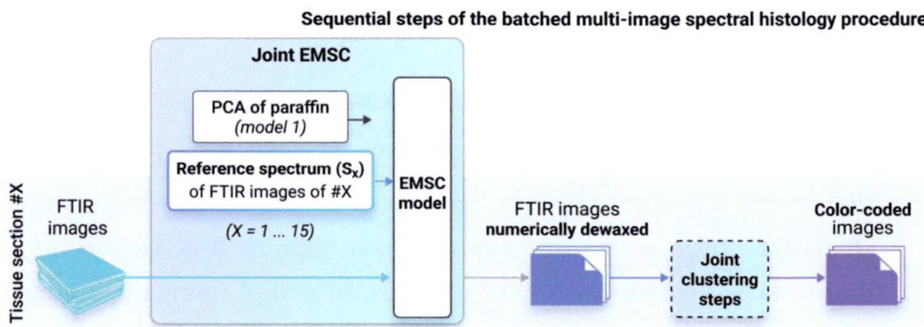

Figure 24: Spectral data processing procedure and protocol

## c)	**Statistical Study**

The proportion of each class derived from the KM for each infrared spectral image was compiled in a database. Sample subgroups were created according to different parameters such as the level of proportion occupied by a class.

Statistical analyses were performed on this digital data using the SPSS® 20 software (IBM, USA).

The continuous variables were analyzed by comparing means using Student's t-test adapted to the distribution.

The discontinuous variables were analyzed using the Chi-square test and Odds Ratios (OR) calculation (a statistical method often used in Epidemiology, expressing the degree of dependency between qualitative random variables).

The alpha risk was fixed at 5%.

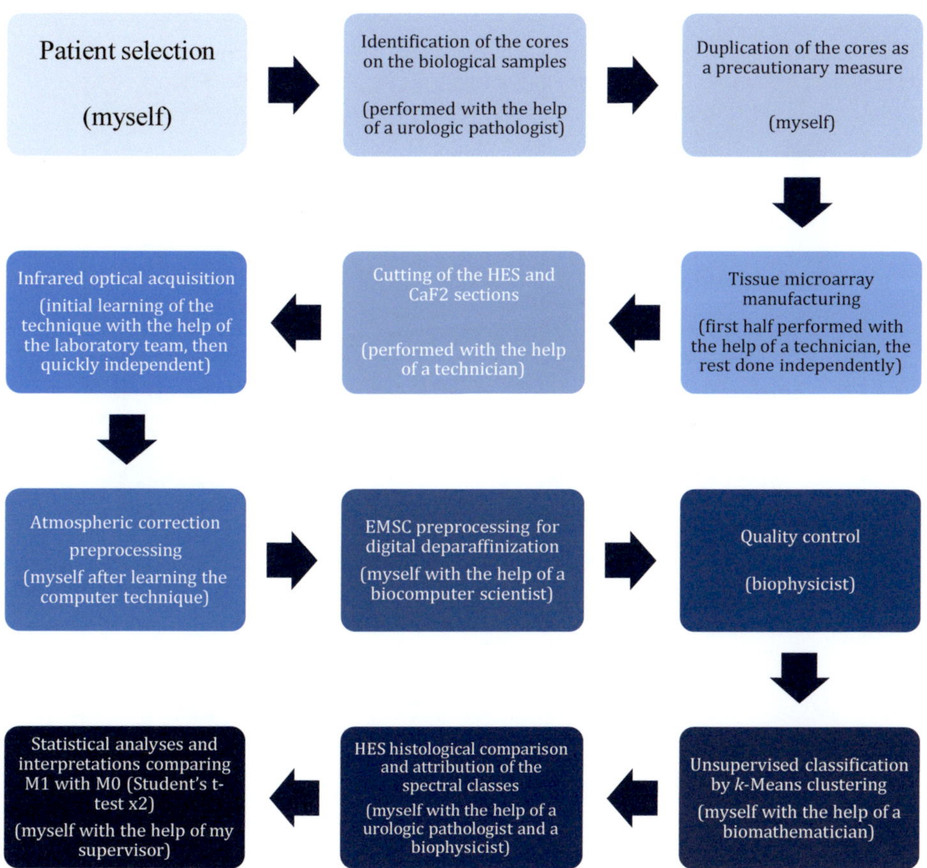

Figure 25: Overview of the materials and methods of the scientific approach

1.7   Results

The clinical, biological, and histological characteristics of the patients included in the study are summarized in Table IV below. The two groups were comparable.

Table IV: Clinical, biological and histological characteristics of the population

	M0 Group n = 50	**M1 Group** n = 50
Age*	67 years (41-81)	69 years (48-79)
Gender	66% men	73% men
Histological Subtype	100% ccRCC**	100% ccRCC
Initial Surgery	100% RNT***	100% RNT
Surgical Margins	100% R0****	100% R0
Targeted Therapy	-	100% Sunitinib
Fuhrman Grade		
1 - 2	56%	52%
3 - 4	44%	48%
Tumor Stage		
T1 - T2	68%	57%
T3 - T4	32%	43%

* Age – Median
** ccRCC: Clear cell renal cell carcinoma
*** RNT: Radical nephrectomy
**** R0. Negative surgical margins

In total 32 cores were missing in the spectral analysis. Optical acquisition was therefore performed on 368 of the 400 initially planned cores.

After the different preprocessing stages, 31 tissue cores with interference were excluded from the definitive analysis for quality control reasons, mainly due to spectral interference that could affect the final attribution of the classes.

Therefore, after the analysis and interpretation stages, a total of 337/400 tissue cores were retained and included for definitive algorithmic and statistical processing (Figure 26).

Preprocessing with the EMSC digital deparaffinization protocol was applied to 337 tissue spectral images along with 13 pure Paraffin spectral images corresponding to the 13 TMA slides.

After deparaffinization, KM classification was performed on all the data simultaneously, i.e., 337 tissue spectral images.

Each spectral image contains around an average 10,000 pixels, i.e., 10,000 unique spectra representing a data set of the developed Big Data Model.

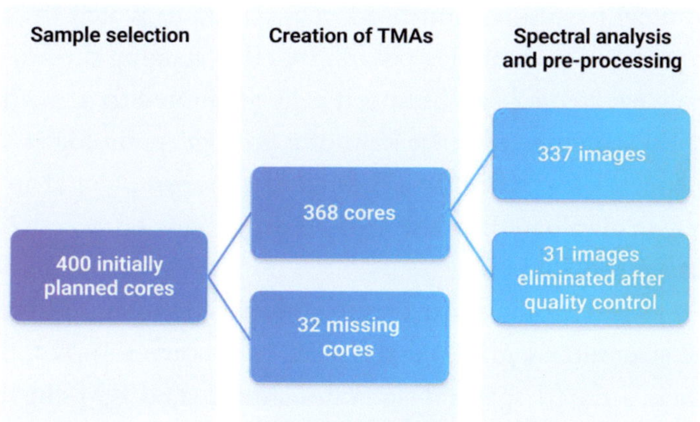

Figure 26: 337 tissue spectral images retained for analysis

Figure 27 shows the distribution of spectral images according to the cores analyzed.

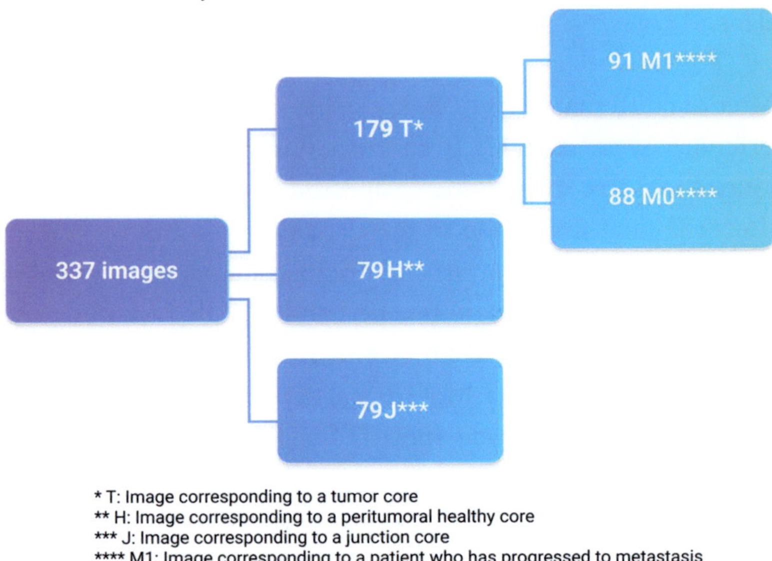

Figure 27: Distribution of spectral images according to the analyzed cores

The KM clustering applied to all the data was used to estimate an optimal partition comprised of 8 classes to which the algorithm randomly attributes colors. By HES staining the adjacent section, each color can be specifically attributed to a given histological structure with the help of a urologic pathologist.

The spectra identified as acquired on the pure Paraffin and therefore eliminated by the EMSC preprocessing protocol are displayed as white pixels.

The revealed results show that it is possible to identify different tissue structures within our renal cell carcinoma samples, based on their infrared spectral signature. Automated KM clustering revealed three clusters corresponding to the tumor zones which are close to the spectral level, as evidenced by the Dendrogram associated with the KM (Figure 28).

This clustering also allowed us to identify a cluster attributed to the connective tissue (cluster no.8, orange color) and a cluster that seems to belong to an inflammatory component (cluster no.2, blue color).

In this clustering, two outlier clusters (no.1 and no.3), corresponding to a small number of pixels positioned on the periphery of the cores (edges), were not considered.

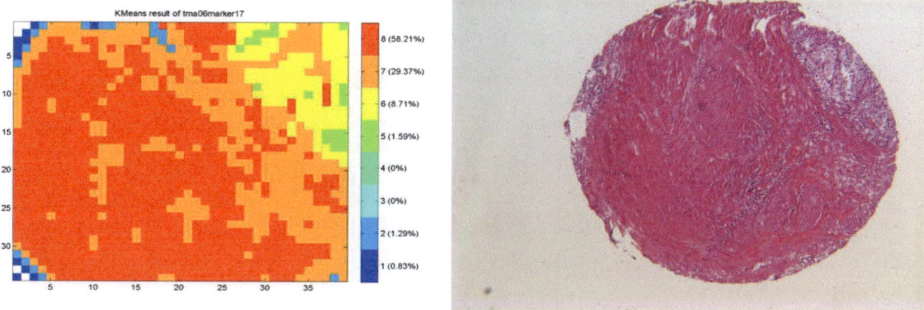

Figure 28: K-means clustering with distribution percentage

We performed a statistical analysis of each class distribution within the spectral images of the non-metastatic (Figure 29) and the metastatic (Figure 30) tumor tissue.

This analysis showed:

The presence of a tumor class (4-turquoise) (Figure 30) appearing as a metastasis risk factor (OR = 2.3 [1.26-4.17]).

Similarly, a class seeming to correspond to an inflammatory cell population (Figure 31) is found to be a metastasis protective factor (OR = 0.5 [0.342-0.815]).

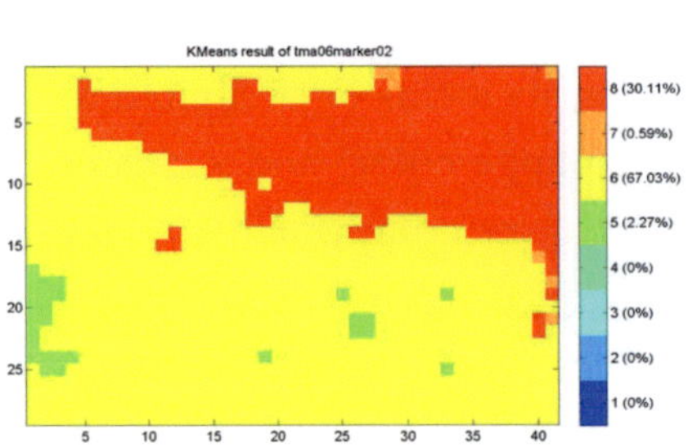 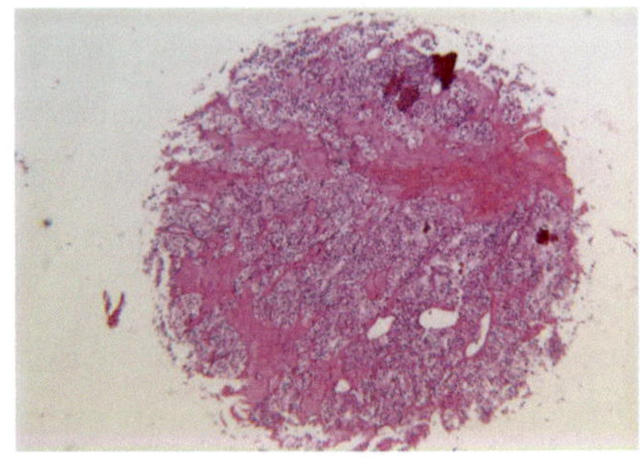

Figure 29: Example KM of a non-metastatic tumor image.
Absence of turquoise cluster no.4

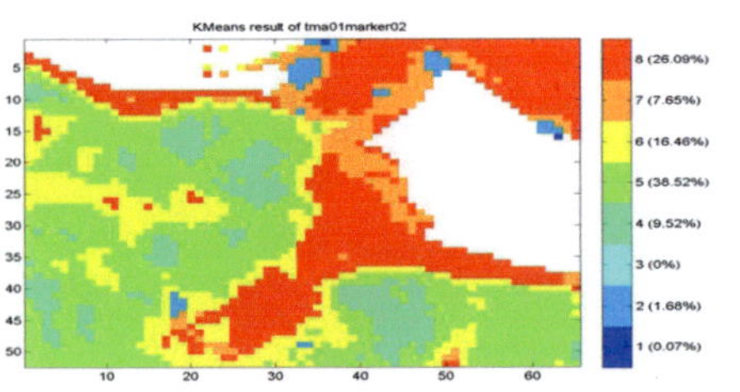 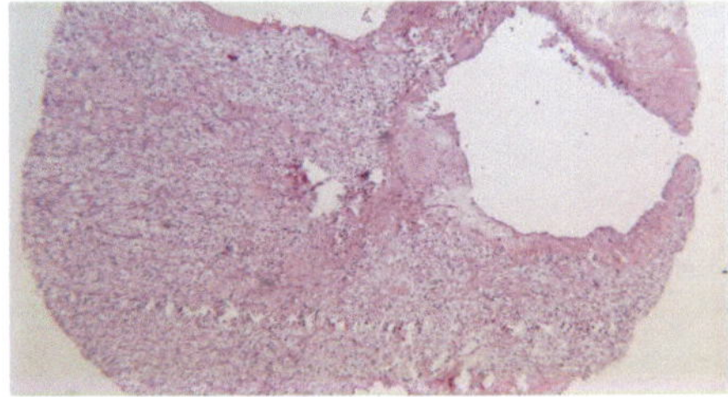

Figure 29: Example KM of a metastatic tumor image with
turquoise cluster no.4 present in the tumor zone

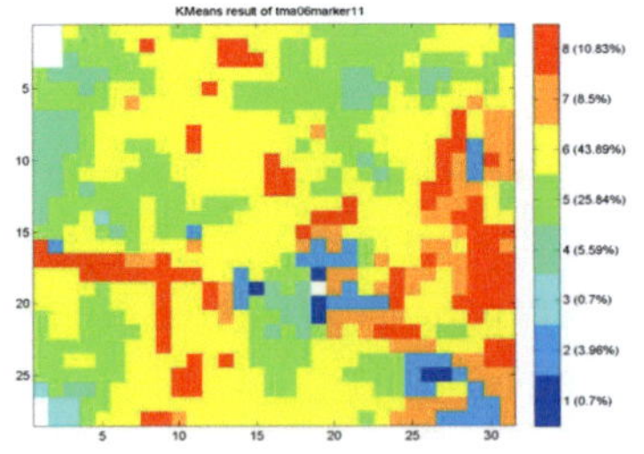 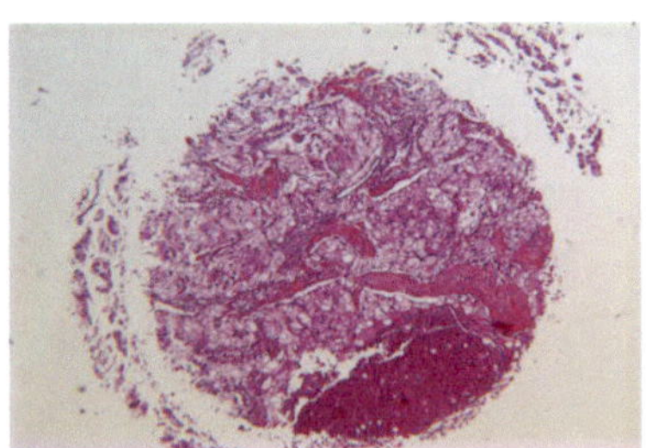

Figure 31: Example KM of a non-metastatic tumor image with blue cluster no.2
present corresponding to what is probably an inflammatory component

The other classes showed no significant result at this stage of
the tests.

The Spectral Signatures of the diverse structures are accessible via the clusters' Centroids, allowing analysis of the characteristic vibration bands.

The Centroid and corresponding Dendrogram therefore represent a Spectral Fingerprint reflecting a Specific Biomolecular Signature (Figure 30).

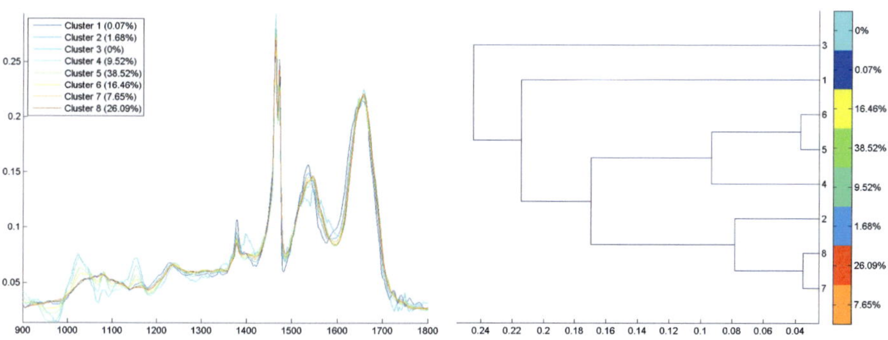

Figure 30: Spectral fingerprint represented by the centroid and its dendrogram

1.8   Discussion

The creation of the methodological approach developed to respond to the problem, which I imagined, designed and actively contributed to in terms of the subject, theme, and method for achieving it, consists in selecting 100 patients with a renal tumor with precise inclusion and exclusion criteria (large cohort compared with the numbers included in other studies of this type in the scientific literature).

These patients are characterized demographically, clinically, biologically, and histologically, then divided into two groups:

One group of metastatic patients and one group of non-metastatic patients with five years of monitoring. The primary tumors of these patients are analyzed by infrared microscopy. The data is preprocessed, then a classification model is created for blind testing.

The spectral histology protocol we followed in this work comprised of three main stages: acquisition of the spectral images, their digital processing, and the allocation of classes to the histological structures. The expected primary outcome was to obtain a classification model that can be used to distinguish renal tumors with a high metastatic risk from those with a low metastatic risk. The two study groups were comparable.

The data acquisition stage was the longest part of this work.

One of the difficulties encountered was inherent to the creation of TMAs because the TMA instrument needle diameter was initially 2 mm, which generated quite large cores causing the recipient Paraffin block to break, which delayed us considerably because we could only produce TMA slides with a maximum of 20 to 30 cores at the start (6 TMAs). This problem was subsequently resolved by the laboratory which ordered a new needle with a more appropriate smaller diameter (1 mm), which allowed us to perform 7 TMAs with between 50 and 80 cores per slide. The diameter of each core in the last 7 TMAs was therefore 1 mm compared with 2 mm for the first 6 TMAs.

It should be noted that systematic duplication of the cores limited data loss in the zones of interest. A total of 32 cores were missing in the spectral analysis; these unavoidable losses of a few cores on each TMA can occur at the different handling stages. I therefore performed the acquisition on a total of 368 of the planned 400 cores.

In Biophotonics, recent scientific literature has shown that the combination of IR spectral imaging with Unsupervised Classification methods like KM can be used to perform spectral histology of human tissues. With this application, the histological structures present in an IR spectral image are differentiated. It makes a comparison between spectral histology and conventional histology possible.

Generally, this method depends on a number of k classes which must be fixed by the user. The choice of the number of k classes therefore becomes difficult when multidimensional data is acquired from a complex sample, like a tissue sample.

In our approach, we used a recent and particularly innovative KM algorithm which can be used to automatically determine the number of k classes using validity indexes to obtain an automated objective spectral histology.

The choice in the standard KM is operator-dependent and therefore arbitrary, hence the potential value of using an automatic KM.

Among the advantages of infrared absorption vibrational spectroscopy is its capacity to characterize and identify the biochemical composition of a fixed and Paraffin-embedded tissue, without extrinsic marking and chemical staining.

It therefore makes it possible to directly analyze a cell or tissue sample in a fast, objective, non-destructive and label-free manner.

Nonetheless, its limitations must also be considered, specifically the fact that lots of spectral data is generated that needs to be validated on several levels. Quality control by a Biophysicist is essential. Several digital processing stages then need to be carried out by a Biomathematician. Lastly, the results must be validated biologically, histologically, and clinically. This work must therefore be carried out within a multidisciplinary team that possesses all these skills.

Immunohistochemical Marking of the cell proliferation mitotic index was performed on the HES slides corresponding to each TMA but could not be exploited in this work.

At present, spectral imaging is a valuable support tool for the real-time diagnosis and in-vitro and in-vivo evaluation of cancerous tissues, since it can be used to establish a specific biomolecular optical signature that is complementary to conventional histopathology.

Other potential applications in Urology could herald a new future for Surgical Oncology, particularly for differentiating malignant or precancerous diseases from benign tumors or in case of doubt concerning intraoperative margins.

As regards the stated results of our current study, they need to be validated by applying a Supervised Classification method to validate our approach. This Supervised Classification method has the advantage of selecting from among the wave numbers, the most discriminating molecular vibrations, which can be represented in the form of spectral bar codes.

<u>Such a method requires</u>:

1) The prior attribution of part of the data to defined classes (connective tissue, metastatic tumor tissue, non-metastatic tumor tissue, inflammation, healthy tissue, etc.). A stage we have just completed during this work.

2) Subsequent validation of the "classifiers" on independent data.

Our completion of TMAs during this work with a sizeable number of different tissues makes it possible to envisage using such an approach with training, internal validation, and test (evaluation on independent samples) data sets.

The spectral marker that seems to relate to inflammation is interesting and appears to be a metastasis protective factor.
This could be explained by a potential stronger local immune response.

Specific attention could also be dedicated to the peritumoral tissue and the marginal zone (Junction) where the availability of Collagen within the Extracellular Matrix and Peritumoral Stroma must be exploited in Spectroscopy, since these areas contain a considerable amount of information.

In particular, we could study the Epithelio-Mesenchymal Transition phenomenon, or try to correlate the Collagen's architectural layout with the evolving metastatic versus the non-metastatic status.

1.9 Conclusion

This study (Figure 33) demonstrates the prognostic potential of infrared microscopy in clear cell renal cell carcinoma. The results are promising. Two optical markers have been identified

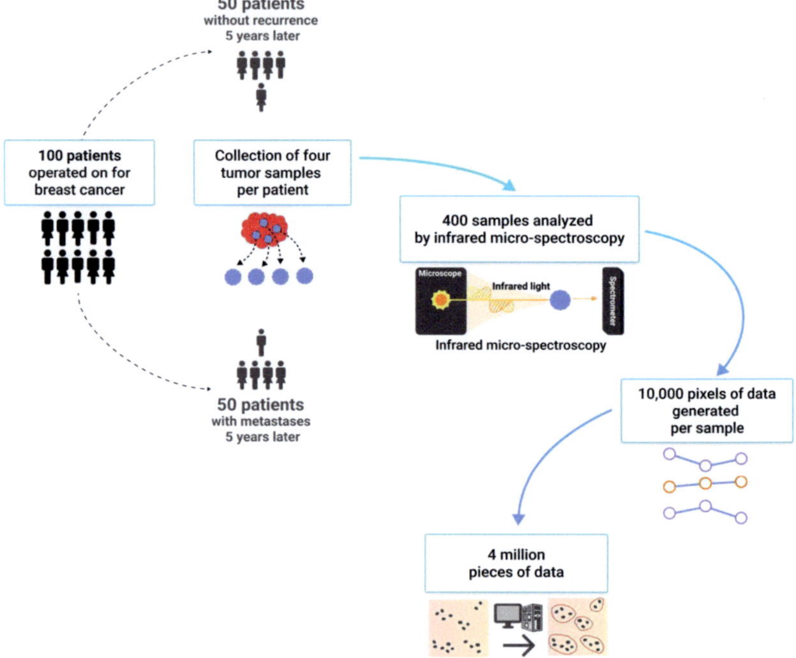

Figure 31: Overview of the study plan

as being linked to the invasive or non-invasive nature of the tumor population with Unsupervised Classification. However, this work will need to be continued to further the investigations and validate this conclusion with Supervised Classification, and by associating these identified spectral markers with histological markers to obtain a Specific Spectral Fingerprint of the metastatic risk that can be used in clinical practice.

1.10   Perspectives

Better knowledge of the prognosis of clear cell renal cell carcinoma can help better define patients requiring surveillance.

As regards the metastatic forms, infrared microscopy data could make it possible to adapt the tyrosine kinase inhibitor treatment, reduce costs and therapeutic resistance and adapt the surveillance frequency. External validation of our prognostic model could prove interesting for future research.

Infrared microscopy also provides an opportunity to study the correlation between pre-operative biopsies and nephrectomy pieces, but also potentially the spectral characterization of the Fuhrman histological grade to improve its accuracy or standardize its interpretation.

Secondly, the continuation of these experiments could aim to:
- <u>Predict</u>, using infrared microscopy, the treatment response to anti-angiogenic targeted therapies, specifically tyrosine kinase inhibitors for metastatic clear cell renal cell carcinoma.
- <u>Compare</u> the spectroscopic data with the Ki67 cell Proliferation Mitotic Index (Anti-MIB1 antibody).

Since the methodology has been developed, we will be able to perform subgroup analyzes as a continuation of this work to study the therapeutic response to Sunitinib, and establish a Spectral Fingerprint and Analysis Algorithm that can be used to predict this response from the outset, and therefore adapt the treatment strategy and sequence, with the knowledge that at present there is no real consensus on the best treatment sequence to adopt for metastatic renal cancer targeted therapies.

The HES sections of the TMAs could be exploited to deepen the Immunohistochemical Analysis on the same slides of the Ki67 Proliferation Mitotic Index, to which the Ploidy Parameter and the PAR-3 cytoplasmic protein could potentially be added.

Lastly, this work could also be applied to other cancers and diseases.

PART FOUR

PROPOSAL AND DEVELOPMENT OF A NEW TECHNOLOGICAL MODEL FOR HEALTH DATA

CASE STUDY TWO: RELYFE® PROJECT

1.11 Introduction

E-Health (Digital Health) encompasses the combined use of new information and communication technologies (NICT) in the health sector. It covers a very diverse range of applications such as Telemedicine, medical devices and connected objects (Internet of Things - IoT), mobile applications, digital platforms, and Artificial Intelligence applied to health data and medical research…

Having observed the lack of data sharing and structuring and the difficulty of applying artificial intelligence to small quantities of data noted in the first study cited in this work relating to predicting metastatic risk in renal cancer, the primary objective of ReLyfe project was to work on the implementation of a new technology architecture for instantly retrieving, sharing and structuring all medical and paramedical health data throughout a patient's care pathway, so it can also be exploited in Artificial Intelligence and research protocols.

The ReLyfe project therefore relates to the development of a secure, universal health profile in the form of a health physical card with a heart-shaped flash-code and a unique identifier (called a Public Key) and/or a digital photo to be saved in a smartphone or retrieved from the Mobile App.
(Figure 34 below, page 88)

This card is connected to an e-health platform (Internet) where health data can be retrieved, filed, structured, and shared securely.

The information in the platform is organized according to a complete care pathway principle, which allows better tracking and identification for both patient and healthcare professional users, including:
- Medical and Surgical History.
- Current Illnesses.
- Laboratory or Radiological Examinations.
- Current Treatments.

The patient must be able to easily connect to a digital interface which uses codes known on the social networks, allowing people who are not familiar with medical terms to learn how to manage their health within a familiar operating environment.

The first technical stage was that of allowing a patient to use this Health Passport to carry on them medical information that is usually very disparate. The patient therefore manages their care pathway and can give the consulting doctor permission to access this information, or they can allow immediate access to vital public data (via the flash-code or Public Key printed on the card) in the event of an emergency.

The patient can access information allowing them to help manage their health on a daily basis, and potentially that of their children or family, including:
- Allergies.
- Screening Examinations.

- Vaccinations.
- Lifestyle Habits.
- Travel.
- Prevention.
- Management of Chronic Diseases.

The two first clearly identified objectives of this e-health big project are therefore the sharing and structuring of health data for the purposes of improved medical collaboration and more effective medical monitoring, which will inevitably lead us to efficient prevention accessible to all, and then to smart and reliable prediction, anywhere in the world.

1.12   Materials and Methods

Patients need a simple tool for the comprehensive management of their health, making them independent and responsible players, with the continued collaboration of their healthcare professionals.

The project was therefore developed with two main focuses:

- Health Data Retrieval, Security, Interoperability, and Structuring.

- Proximity, sharing and a simple and direct (peer-to-peer) connection with all medical and paramedical healthcare professionals.

To achieve this, I created a start-up company first called InnovHealth® in April 2016 and then ReLyfe Group in April 2021. It was registered in the Reims Trade and Companies Register ("RCS") under number: 818 991 929. Its legal form is a "Société par Actions Simplifiée" [Simplified Joint Stock Company] ("SAS"). The seed funding for the start-up and the various research and development programs was provided initially by the French Public Investment Bank "Bpifrance", health professionals associates and other private investors. The technological development required the recruitment of a team of ten full-time engineers and developers in the early days, which later grew to over twenty. The technical procedures were divided into two parts: ReLyfe PATIENT (patient-dedicated card and platform) and ReLyfe PRO (access for healthcare professionals, researchers, clinics, hospitals and primary healthcare providers and centers). These two parts were developed in two stages. The responsive ReLyfe PATIENT platform to which the card is connected was developed between 2016 and 2020. The responsive ReLyfe PRO platform was developed between 2018 and 2022. The two platforms are closely linked, use a hybrid technology architecture (several integrated technologies and languages) and are both accessible via the web or via the iOS and Android stores. The model was based on a "two-sided" interaction inspired by the "two-sided market" platform model described by winner of the 2014 French Nobel Prize for Economic Sciences Professor Jean Tirole (see below).

A.   Health Data Extraction and Structuring

Thanks to the developed technology model, patients can instantly retrieve and file their health data. They save them in a secure digital safe which has strong two-factor authentication, for a comprehensive and hierarchized view throughout their life.

They integrate them either by themselves (or via their healthcare professional) by entering data from databases validated according to the WHO international standards, in particular the International Classification of Diseases (ICD-10), the VIDAL international medication database, then the structuring is involved automatically via the integrated artificial intelligence model that classifies documents and extracts from them the pertinent information (see below).

B.   Information Adoption and Sharing via the Patient

Now is a particularly opportune time to digitize the care pathway. The measures proposed by the French Government under the health system reform called "Ma Santé 2022" [My Health

2022] are prompting the emergence of new ideas, particularly for the management of health information.

> "The most delicate issue on which we focused in UX (User Experience) is the difference of language used by patients (according to their level of comprehension and literacy) and practitioners (initiated in the medical scientific language) to have structured technical and usable data. It must be easily entered and understandable by both parties and scientifically exploitable by the AI. We had to adapt each side of the platform to the identified needs of the users, both at the level of the verbatim and at the level of the possible actions according to their relevance to have an optimized and efficient data structuring."
>
> *Quote by Jane Seneor, ReLyfe Head of Product Design*

According to the 2018 and 2019 Deloitte barometers, patients are prepared to spend and invest an average of €29 per month for a quality, personalized service focused on their health. They are also completely happy (85%) to share their data online.

The platform we developed in this project is primarily supplied with information by the patient who owns the card, under very strict conditions:

- Either by entering information directly from databases created by us for this purpose based on validated references and with the help of a dedicated search engine.

For diseases, we use the ICD 10 which has been revised and simplified for better patient accessibility.
For drugs, we use the VIDAL database which has been implemented for patients, again to facilitate accessibility.

This solution, which aims to structure information around dedicated databases, will also allow easier use of the data produced.

- Or by scanning results from reports obtained in file format (PDF or other, all formats are accepted) directly (drag and drop technique by clicking the mouse on the file concerned), or with the help of a Plug-Link technology, which is represented by an integrated Virtual Printout (which we developed in a C/C++ low-level computer language then connected directly to the ReLyfe platform's architecture, with structuring of the data sent), followed by automated exploitation of the content by OCR (see below).

- Or by photographing an image: Dermatological lesion or other clinical photos (ReLyfe PRO function currently being used at the Plastic Surgery Department of Tenon Hospital within the Paris Hospitals "Assistance Publique - Hôpitaux de Paris / AP-HP") for monitoring pre-and post-operative scars, for instance, or dermatological follow-up.

C. Universal Digital Medical Identity

A unique and personal digital identity has been devised and implemented with the use of a heart-shaped modified QR-Code. This new flash-code is printed on the phygital card (Figure 34). Phygital means using technology to link the digital world to the physical world. Hence the name: phy(sical)(di)gital.
The objective is clear: to offer the user a unique interactive experience by combining the physical and the digital experience.

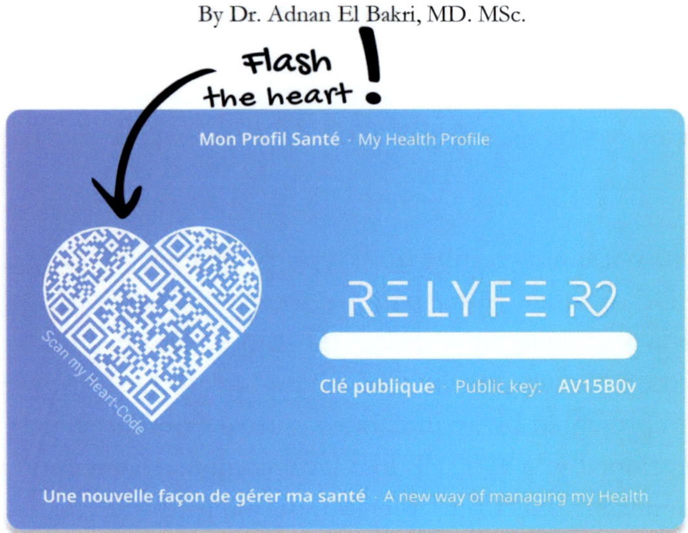

Figure 32: Personal health card in digital format

Each card has a secure and non-duplicable identity. This flash-code is correlated with a public personal 7-character key associated with the flash-code (the virtual card key begins with VIR) and therefore belonging to each card. Either the patient is automatically assigned a personal virtual card by creating an account on the platform and requests a corresponding physical card, or they receive a physical card from their practitioners that will be mirrored as a digital card when they register. A card can only be linked to a single account. A single account cannot have two cards except for children's accounts which are attached to the two profiles of the two parents.

These two elements: the flash code and the key, provide strong identification, traceability elements and interoperability elements. It should be noted that no health data is stored physically on this card which represents only an access key.
If the card is lost, it is simply dissociated from the account in the corresponding section of the platform.

D. Method of Accessing Personal and Family Medical Information

Within this project, we also developed "family" access, i.e., a shared space allowing each parent to access not only their own personal health data, but that of each of their children for pediatric monitoring, which is instantly updated directly on the two parents' two cards.

For each item of information entered in the platform, each patient can decide:

Whether this information is part of their emergency profile, i.e., accessible to everyone in any situation.

Whether this information is under their responsibility, i.e., they decide themselves (or their trusted person decides) who can access it (total or partial access).

The "Emergency Profile" with public access, can be accessed with a simple scan of the flash-code using any mobile telephone (via the camera function) (Figure 35, access procedure).

In the event of an accident, for example, this instant access gives practitioners immediate access to essential vital data for their treatment.

Each patient can give medical and paramedical practitioners access to their information via strong, unique and temporary authentication (temporary access), or by associating them directly with their account as appointed healthcare professionals (permanent access).

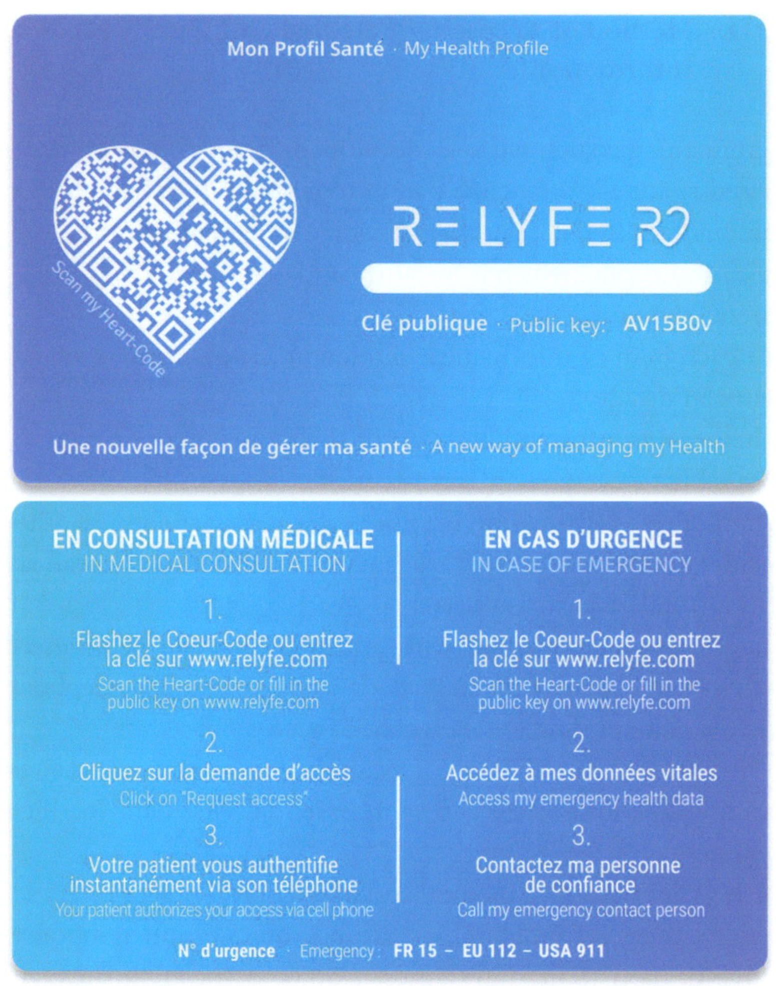

Figure 33: Front and back of the ReLyfe health card with the access procedure

The menu and interface of the ReLyfe PATIENT and PRO platform are presented in Figure 36 & 37.

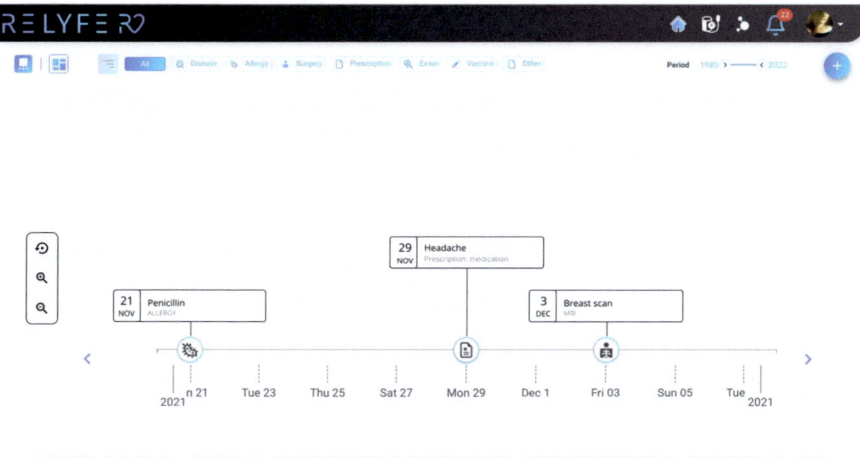

*Figure 34: Menu and interface of the ReLyfe PATIENT platform
(collaborative and interactive timeline)*

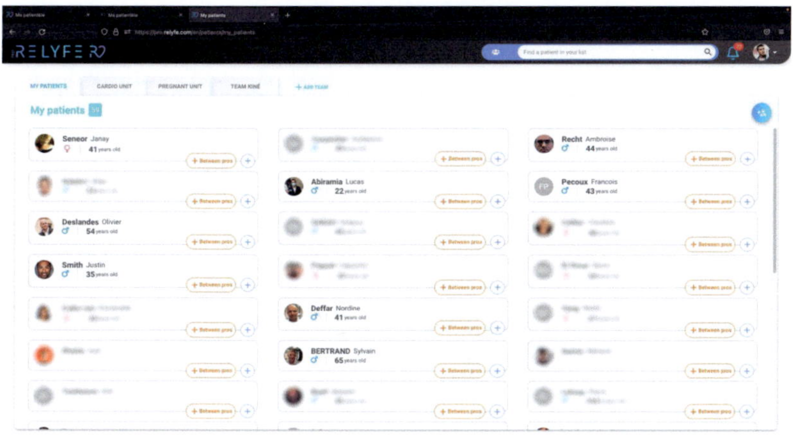

Figure 35: Menu and interface of the ReLyfe PRO platform

1.13   Technology Platform Developed within the Project

A.   Design of the Database and Global Technical Architecture

The global database (Table V, page 98) was designed according to the following information and criteria, which required setting up a new, considered, hybrid, flexible and universal technological construction.

First of all, the development of a comprehensive, personal, interactive digital health record via a card, which is 100% interoperable with all existing IT systems and business software in the world, based on a modern vision which allows patients to directly retrieve and manage their health data, and allows healthcare professionals and researchers to make easier use of this information in research protocols.

The platform also needed to be designed so that it could structure the information as it was received, for the successful implementation and practice of algorithmic medicine.

Several sections were then determined straight away within the platform all linked to a patient's care timeline (Figure 36):
-    Medical and Surgical History.
-    Allergies.
-    Medical Consultations.
-    Treatments.
-    Biological Examinations / Imaging.
-    Measurements.
-    Lifestyle.

<u>Patients</u> must be able to share their health information through a structured timeline with their healthcare professionals via:

- A configurable public profile.
- Sharing options that allow you to share some document(s) or your entire profile (dynamically updated) with a practitioner or a care team via direct ReLyfe network sharing (for which the patient can define the duration), the display of a flashable Heart-Code® or via a link that can be copied into any sharing, email, or chat application.
- A request for access to complete or partial data with an authorization system that uses a signature link sent by SMS or email to a mobile device.
- A dedicated care team with whom they can communicate (send healing photos, add comments or receive video calls initiated by the professionals).

<u>Healthcare Professionals</u> need a dedicated interface to communicate with their patients and follow them efficiently by accessing their ReLyfe profiles and timelines, to add information about them, receive in real-time any information, reports, examinations, or biological results added by their patients, colleagues or third parties, but above all to be able to collaborate with their peers:

- List of patients appointed to each doctor or to care teams they belong to.
- List of the care teams they are part of.
- Communication tools to easily exchange with the patient or their teams, refer a patient to a colleague or seek a second opinion.
- Consultation system with report generation at the end.
- Electronic treatment prescription system.
- Virtual printing module or driver allowing documents generated via the doctors' third-party software to be easily and

securely sent directly from this software to their patients' ReLyfe timeline.

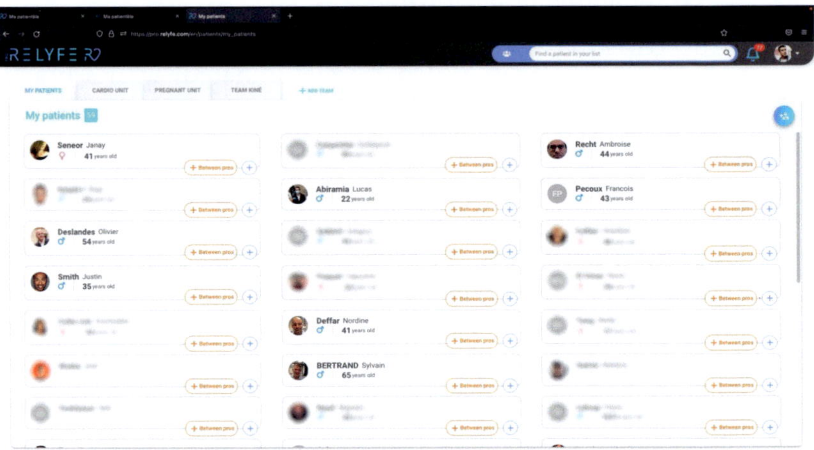

Figure 36: Create lists of care teams in the ReLyfe PRO platform

<u>Healthcare Centers</u> must have dedicated access:
- Chronic disease monitoring.
- List of care teams in the facility and the ability to create new ones and add staff by care team (Figure 38).
- Photographic monitoring system for dermatological problems or post-operative scar follow-up.
- Management of the activation of cards connected with the facility.
- Administrative management of patients connected with the hospital or clinic.

B. Collaboration Technology & Architecture

This platform offers three major collaboration ways responding to the actual health professional needs:

- <u>Collaboration within a care team</u> in the form of a private chat that also allows video calls (to the team or team members individually), private care protocols template creation and images or administrative documents to be shared (Figure 39).

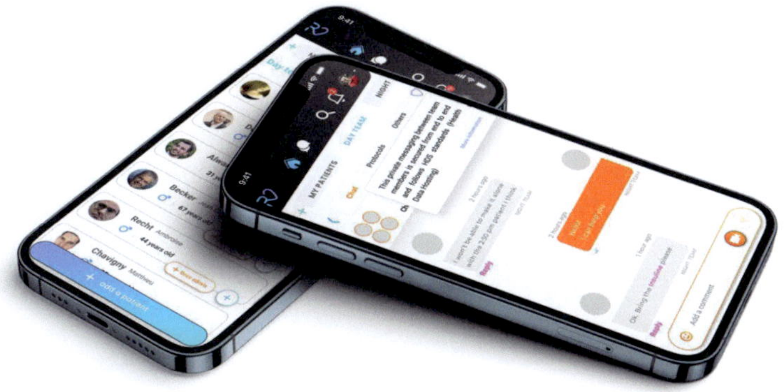

Figure 37: Private communication within a care team

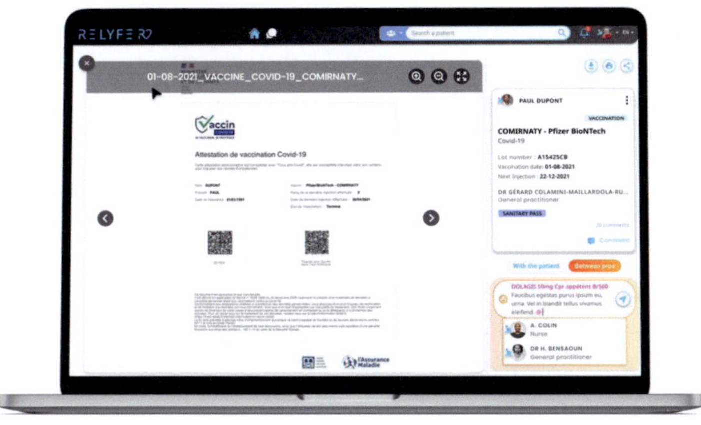

Figure 38: Collaboration with the patient and/or between health professionals on a medical data

<u>Collaboration around medical data, with the patient or between professionals</u>: a comment component allowing the structured mention of drugs (linked to the VIDAL database) or any health professional who has shared access to this data. These comments are linked to this specific medical data, with or without document, and accessible to any professional invited to consult it (Figure 38).

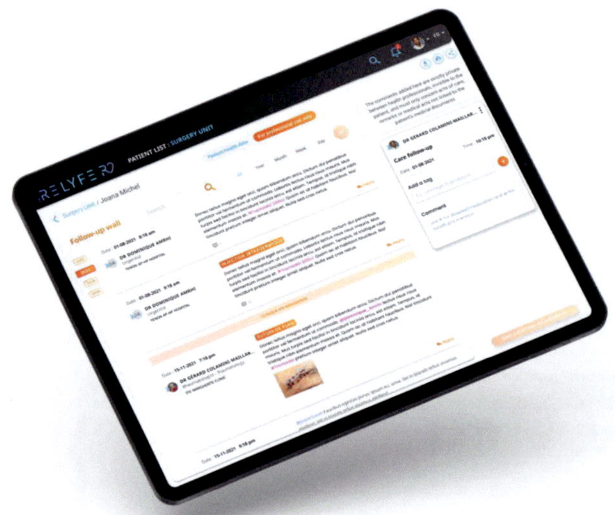

Figure 39: Collaboration around a patient with a "patient wall"

- <u>Collaboration around a patient</u> with a "Patient Wall" that chronologically follows the patient throughout his life. Accessible to any healthcare professional currently linked with the patient, this wall shows an aggregation of all past and present professional exchanges around the patient (except for the content of the private care team chat): comments exchanged on the data, private imagery taken with ReLyfe PRO, completed care protocols and any other information to be entered directly. A powerful search engine allows to sort and filter any relevant information (Figure 39).

This architecture will allow the different stakeholders within a healthcare system to interconnect around the patient's health platform by efficiently sharing information and creating a unique data flow (Figure 40).

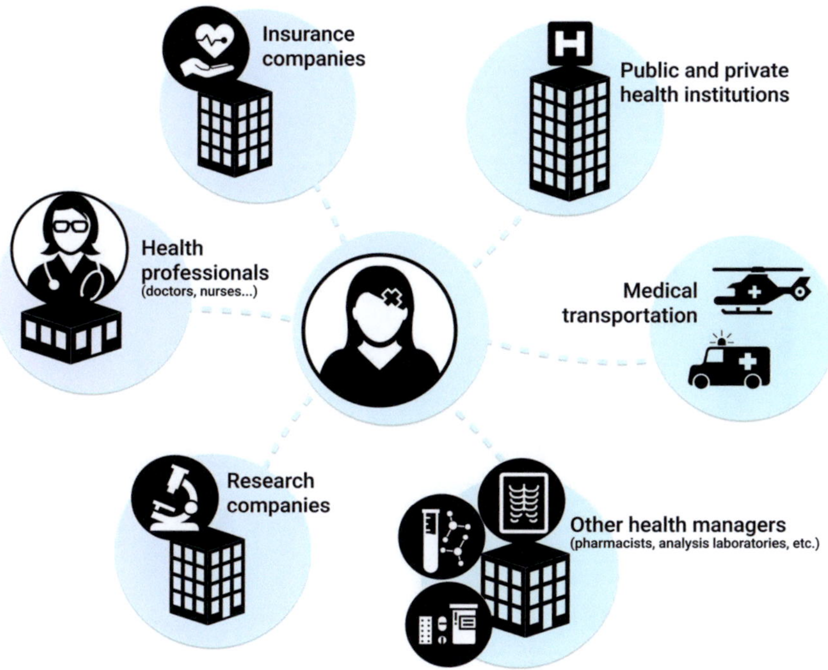

Figure 40: Interconnection of the different health stakeholders

By Dr. Adnan El Bakri, MD. MSc.

Table V: Computer construction of the database foundational architecture

The whole system is connected to an interactive telecommunication tool allowing the platform to perform telemedicine (teleconsultation, tele-assessment), with no specific installation constraints, hence the need to use only the Internet. Our communication platform uses Jitsi API (Application Programming Interface) which is HDS/GDPR/HIPAA compliant. Jitsi is seamlessly integrated into our platform and benefits from the data that the patient shares during a call allowing real-time collaborative medical video consultations or follow-up without the constraints of installing additional software or applications.

API relies on a triangular then peer-to-peer architecture in which a central server is used to put patients (Client A in Figure 41) and healthcare professionals (Client B in Figure 41) in contact with one another who want to exchange media or data flows without other intermediaries (Figure 41).

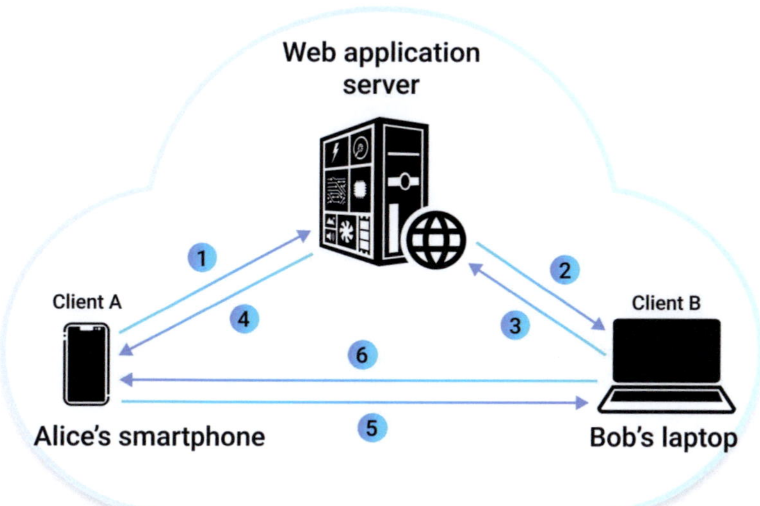

Figure 41: Triangular data exchange architecture

Lastly, an emergency public profile is accessible by flashing the Heart-Code or entering the Public Key of the patient's card.

It allows access to vital shared patient information in the event of an accident or loss of consciousness (faintness or coma, for example). Through this page there's a function that allows the unlock of the patient's ReLyfe data by sending an SMS to be instantly validated:

- by the patient himself (e.g., in the case of a consultation with a non-ReLyfer professional).

- by one of the contacts previously filled in by the patient who has de facto the authorization to give access to the patient's ReLyfe timeline.

C. Choice of the Techniques Used

The ReLyfe complex program and architecture was developed using several hybrid modern technologies (Figure 42):

- <u>Python/FastApi</u>: A framework known for its easy integration for Artificial Intelligence and declarative APIs.
- <u>Node.js/Express</u>: Used as our gateway to distribute all the web and mobile demands to the needed microservices, our security layer passes by it and enables fine tuning the authentication and authorization based on roles (Healthcare Professional, Patient, Guest…).
- <u>PHP/Symfony</u>: used for its MVC -Model-View-Controller- architecture in some of our back microservices.
- <u>JavaScript/React</u>: Used for our web applications, enables highly reactive interactions, and divides the application into reusable components.

- <u>Capacitor</u>: A wrapper to transform our web application into a mobile app (Android and iOS) to benefit from using the phone's peripherals.
- <u>React Native</u>: A React-based mobile application framework used by healthcare professionals that focuses on maximizing the use of the camera.

Python is a high-level, general-purpose programming language. Its design philosophy emphasizes code readability with the use of significant indentation. Its language constructs and object-oriented approach aim to help programmers write clear, logical code for small- and large-scale projects.

FastAPI is a modern, fast (high-performance), web framework for building APIs, it is known for being fast, robust, and intuitive, making it easy to handle fast iterations.

PHP is an open-source programming language mainly used to produce dynamic web pages via a **HTTP** (Hypertext Transfer Protocol) server. HTTP is a client-server communication protocol developed for the World Wide Web (WWW).
HTTPS (S for Secure) is the variant used for secure protocols. The most widely known HTTP clients are web browsers that allow a user to access a server containing data.
PHP can also function as any locally interpreted language; in all cases it is an object-oriented imperative language. PHP has been used to create many famous websites like Facebook and Wikipedia. It is considered one of the foundations for the creation of so-called dynamic websites, but also web applications.
The initial choice for our POC was the CakePHP framework for its Object-Relational Mapping (ORM) power.

It is an open-source web framework, distributed under the Massachusetts Institute of Technology (MIT) license. It follows the **MVC** design pattern, which is a software architecture pattern intended for graphical interfaces.

We switched to a React web application and React Native mobile app to separate front- and back-end for production and scalability in 2019.

Symfony, created in 2005, is a set of PHP components and an open-source MVC framework written in PHP. It provides modulable and adaptable functionalities that facilitate and speed up a website's development.

React is an open-source JavaScript software library developed by Facebook since 2013. The main aim of this library is to facilitate the creation of single-page web applications via the creation of state-dependent components and generating a HTML page (or portion) with each state change. This library only generates the application interface, considered as the view in the MVC model. It is distinguished from its competitors by its flexibility and performance. Amongst others, it is used by Netflix, Yahoo, Airbnb, Sony and the Facebook teams.

HTML is a HyperText Markup Language created in 1992 in open-source format designed to represent web pages. It is a language that can be used to write hypertext, hence its name.

It can also be used to semantically and logically structure and format page content, and include multimedia resources such as images, data entry forms and computer programs.

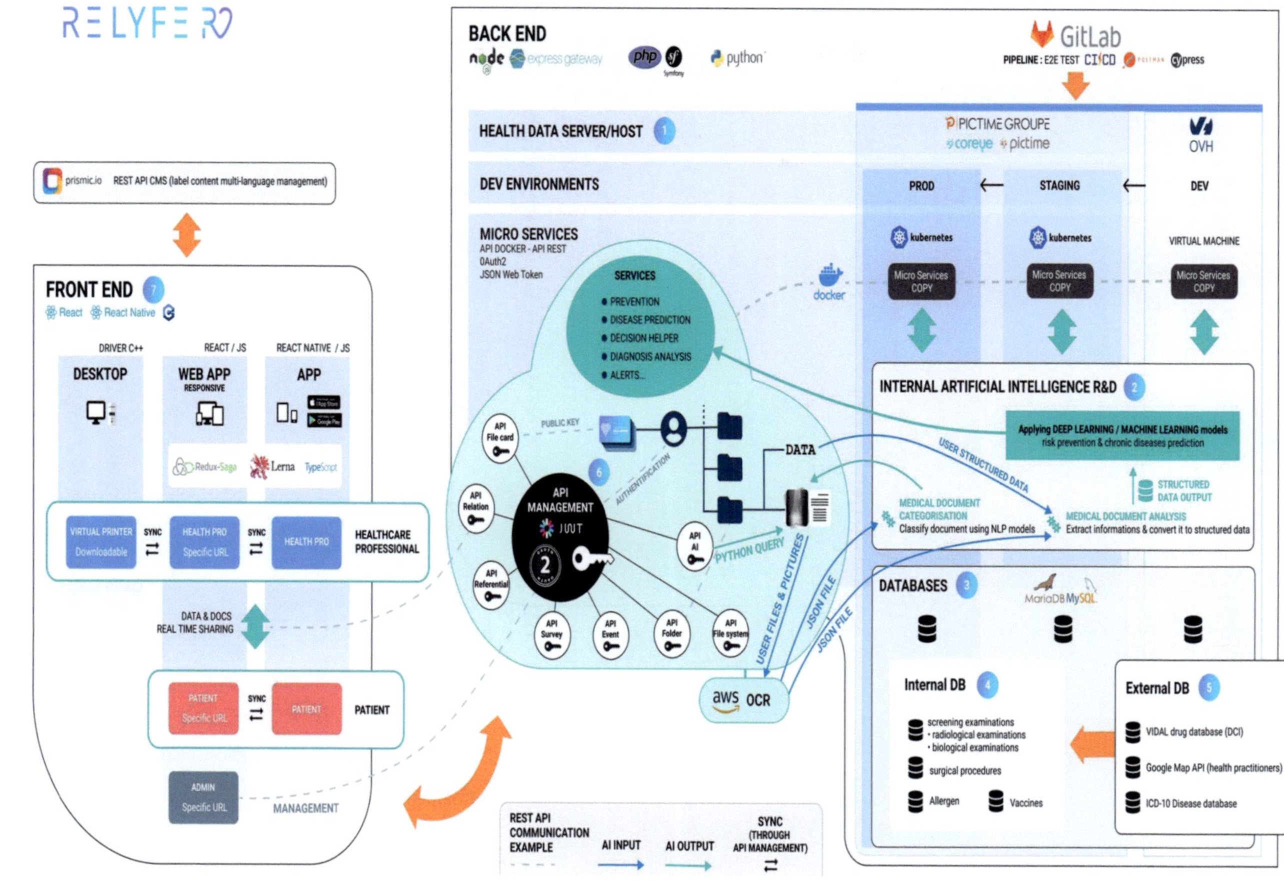

Figure 42: Technical environment, technologies, systems and servers used

It can be used to create documents that are interoperable with a great variety of equipment in line with the web's accessibility requirements. It is often used together with programming language JavaScript and Cascading Style Sheets (CSS).

CSS is a computer language which describes the presentation of HTML and XML documents. The standards defining CSS are published by the World Wide Web Consortium (W3C).
It was introduced in 1996 and is now routinely used in website design and is currently well supported by web browsers.

JavaScript, created in 1995, is a computer programming language mainly used in interactive web pages, but also for servers. Along with the HTML and CSS technologies, JavaScript is considered one of the Internet's core technologies. A large majority of websites use it, and most web browsers have a dedicated JavaScript engine for interpreting it.

Capacitor is an open-source native runtime for building web native applications. Create cross-platform iOS, Android, and Progressive Web Apps with JavaScript, HTML, and CSS, it allows us to embed our web code to publish the mobile app as a native to the stores.

React Native is an open-source mobile applications framework created by Facebook.
It is used to develop applications for Android, iOS (Google and Apple smartphone operating systems) by enabling developers to use React with the native functions of these platforms.

Node.js is a backend JavaScript framework. One of the reasons Node.js frameworks are a popular choice for developers building a flexible and scalable backend is its event-driven, non-blocking nature. To use Node.js together with React.js (both use JavaScript) make code scalable and highly efficient, for real-time data management or streaming (highly recommended for a constant server connection), for high server load (help in handling requests and maintaining server load balance), for JSON APIs (reusability of the code enables sharing within React.js), for robust backend, lightweight app and asynchronous data loading through callback functions, for bundles of applications to simplify the compilation process. Both React and Node.js happen to have different functions in the web development process but can be used together to reap multiple benefits. Node.js is used by several tech-giants like Netflix, PayPal etc.

Prismic is an API-based headless CMS (Content Management System), backend tool that provides a very solid architectural foundation and allows us easily managing, storing, and modeling of the web app and app content (for instance all interface page titles, texts and field labels) in one place, and providing translation and localization for different languages. Even better, it allows marketing and content staff to iterate the texts without having a developer needed. It comes with a React package, and so provides a React integration to fetch and display our content that includes special components for rendering structured fields. To render Rich Text, for instance, we can use:

```
<PrismicRichText field={document.data.example_title} />
```

The ReLyfe platform has also been connected to the VIDAL database via its dedicated API interface, making it possible to extract the drugs available in France and all the ICD-10 information.

The mobile application uses the React-Native technology.

The mobile application uses the ReLyfe REST (Representational State Transfer, see below) API to extract and transmit health data to the platform.

The virtual printer was developed in C/C++ language and uses the REST API to transmit the documents, files and images generated by healthcare professionals to ReLyfe.

This Multi-Technology Global Architecture, together with the devised complex data exchange and interoperability mechanisms, are illustrated in Figure 43. It served as the basis for the IT technical development and understanding of the various interactions envisaged.

This hybrid new innovative concept has been registered and protected by copyright and trademark rights in the 150 signatory countries of the Bern Convention, and protected by intellectual property rights: the "Institut National de la Propriété Industrielle" [National Industrial Property Institute] ("INPI") in France, the European Union Intellectual Property Office (EUIPO) in Europe, the United States Patent and Trademark Office (USPTO) in the United States and the "Organisation Africaine de la Propriété Intellectuelle" [African Intellectual Property Organization] ("OAPI") in Africa.

The computer source code was filed and protected with the "Agence de Protection des Programmes" [Program Protection Agency] ("APP") in France as an original piece of software; this can also be used to specify and confirm the creation date.

It was also filed with the "Société des Gens De Lettres" [French Authors Society] ("SGDL") which supports writers and defends their rights.

D. Authentication and Authorization

Authentication is done with the JWT Standard.

Basically, the user is given a token that contains his identification and role. The token expires in a short period and the user has a refresh token to get another one.

By using this technique, we can revoke access to a user if we detect suspicious activity or if the original token is compromised.

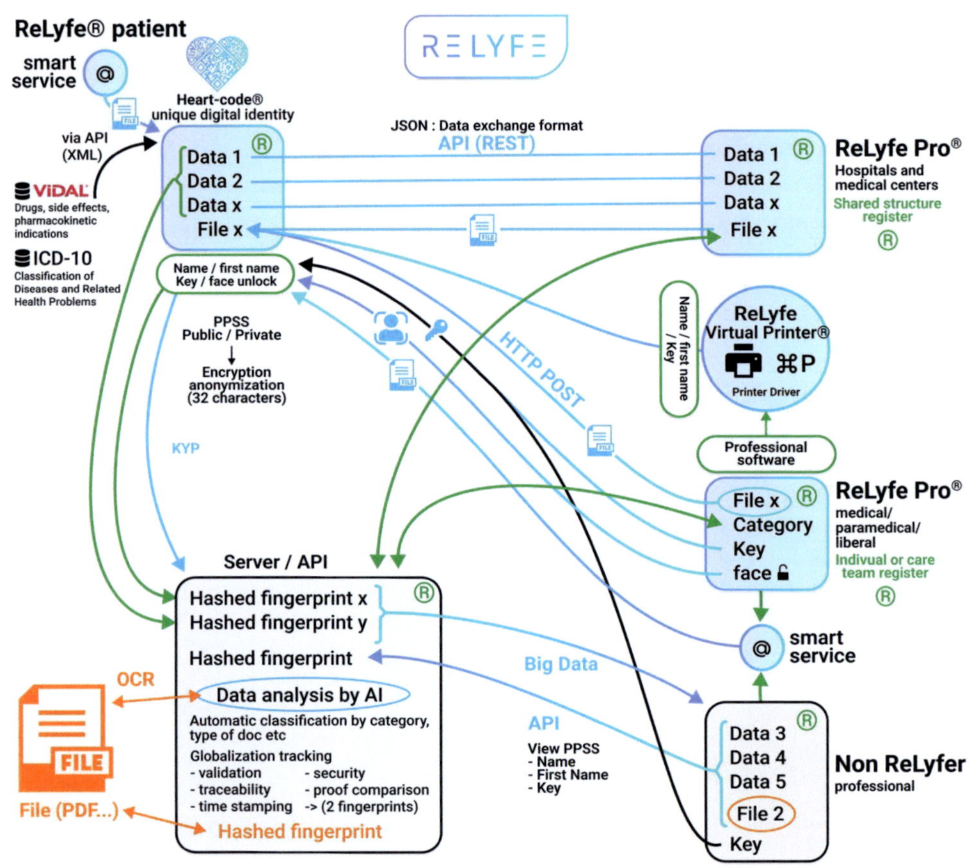

Figure 43: Global technology architecture, interoperability and data exchange

E. Interoperability and API Management Method Implemented

In IT, an API is a standardized set of classes, methods, functions, and constants which serves as a frontend by which software offers services to other software (Figure 44).

It is offered by a software library or web service, most often accompanied by a description which specifies how "consumer" programs can make use of the "supplier" program's functions.

In the contemporary software industry, computer applications use many programming interfaces, and programming is done by reusing function blocks provided by third-party software.

This assembly construction requires the programmer to know how to interact with the other software, which depends on their programming interface.

a)   Smart ReLyfe Services

We have developed multiple services that are technology improvement for efficiency or authentication.

1. Smart Face Authentication

In response to the imperative need for international organizations like UNHCR to be able to authenticate the medical data of refugees who do not have a smartphone or email address (as it was mandatory to create a ReLyfe account and authenticate until now), we have developed a way to recognize somebody at 99.9% from a first photo of him/her, with an AI comparison algorithm when taking a second photo with a smartphone camera.

In concrete terms, this will allow healthcare practitioners to immediately access the ReLyfe profiles of refugees simply by scanning their face at the beginning of a medical consultation. This solution can be implemented to optimize other use cases, especially for people with low agility or digital access, those using assistive technology or accessibility in general (illiteracy, illectronism, with disabilities, etc.).

This allows for real-time identification of an individual without the need to enter personal data, a usually time-consuming and error-prone step.

2. Smart Instant Integration Mailing Upload

A smart dual system for uploading health documents, simple and fast, to gain efficiency.

For the patient via his email registered in ReLyfe, to be able to send a document directly in his timeline without opening ReLyfe via *smart@relyfe.com*. The document will be then scanned by our AI and structured accordingly to its extracted content.

Similarly, for the healthcare professional to be able to directly add a document to a patient's timeline via email using the patient's Public Key on the *<patient_public_key>@relyfe.com* model (Figure 44).

This last system can also be used with non-ReLyfers professionals from anywhere in the world. To be more convenient, the patient can give his personal email *<patient_public_key>@relyfe.com* to any health professional worldwide, so any type of health document or image communicated to the patient will be automatically recognized, securely integrated, and directly structured in his timeline.

Smart@ReLyfe is an SMTP listener that will handle all mails received, considering the attachment, the body, and the subject, and can understand for who to add the document and when. Our AI algorithm is also integrated with this service to automatically detect the type of the document and extract prescriptions or examinations if needed, in order to personalize the treatment and medication compliance for example (alerts).

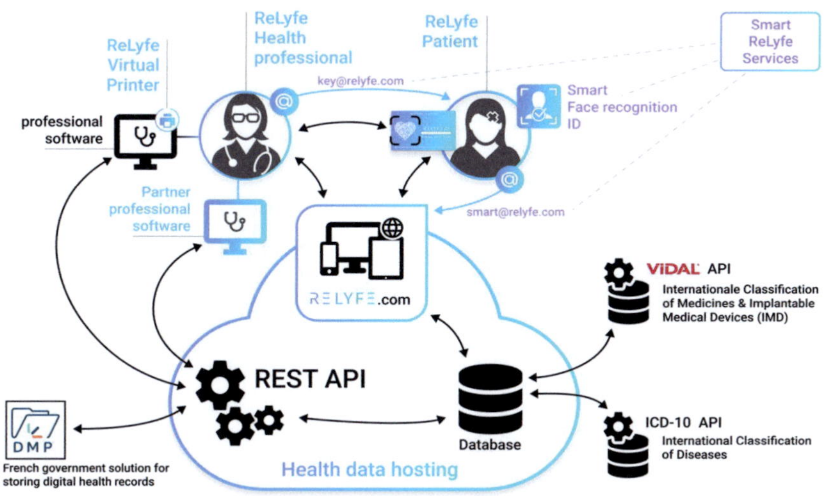

Figure 44: Interoperability and different interactions developed in ReLyfe

The programmer does not need to know the details of the third-party software's internal logic, and this is not generally documented by the supplier. Software like operating systems, database management systems, programming languages and application servers have their own programming interfaces.

F.   The REST Software Architectural Style of our Coded API

REST is a software architecture style that defines a set of constraints to be used to create web services. Web services that conform to the REST architecture style, also called RESTful web services, establish interoperability between computers (Figure 45).

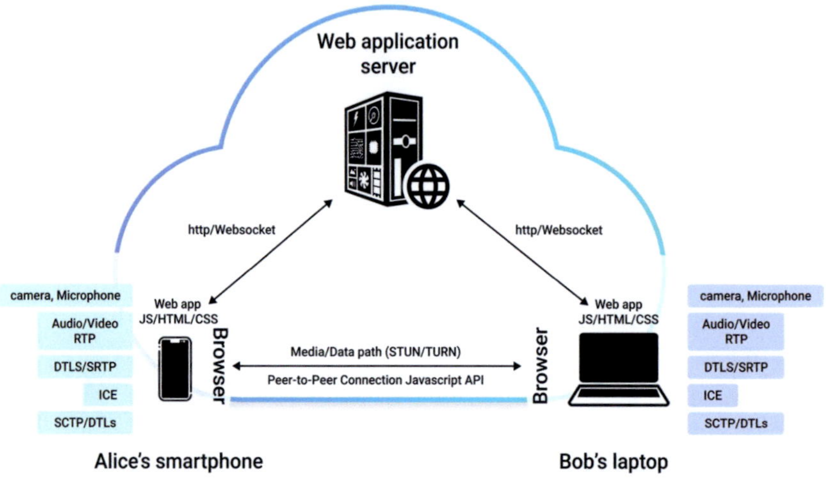

Figure 45: Exchanges and interactions between different applications on the Internet

The REST web services allow the systems carrying out searches to handle web resources via their textual representations through a series of predefined uniform operations.

Web resources were first defined on the World Wide Web (www) as documents or files identified by their web address (URL for Uniform Resource Locator).

However, they now have a much more generic and abstract definition which includes any thing or entity that can be identified, named, addressed, or managed in any way on the web.

In a REST web service, searches carried out on the URL of a resource produce a response whose body is formatted in

HTML, Extensible Markup Language (XML), JavaScript Object Notation (JSON) or another format.

XML and JSON are important interoperability elements.

G. Artificial Intelligence Built-in Data Structuring Algorithm with Deep Learning

Structuring medical data in the world remains a big challenge because of the lack of health data for privacy reasons and the lack of methods and approaches on processing several languages and standards. Few of those challenges are classifying the health documents and extracting the drug-related information and the biological parameters from the medical prescription and biological examinations (blood tests for example) respectively. To our knowledge, over the last decade, there are less than five theoretical research projects on structuring medical documents. In ReLyfe, we have proposed a new functionality for extracting drug-related information from clinical scanned documents while respecting patients' privacy. In addition, we have developed a new service for structuring biological parameters from biological results. Moreover, these functionalities have been deployed in our production platform and are already used by patients and professionals. We have closed a gap between the theoretical and practical work by creating the ReLyfe application adapted to real-life constraints. These services can be implemented on any web or mobile platform. They are based on the combination of a Rule-Based System and a Deep Learning approach. The global objective was to obtain an intelligent system capable of recognizing all medical semantics

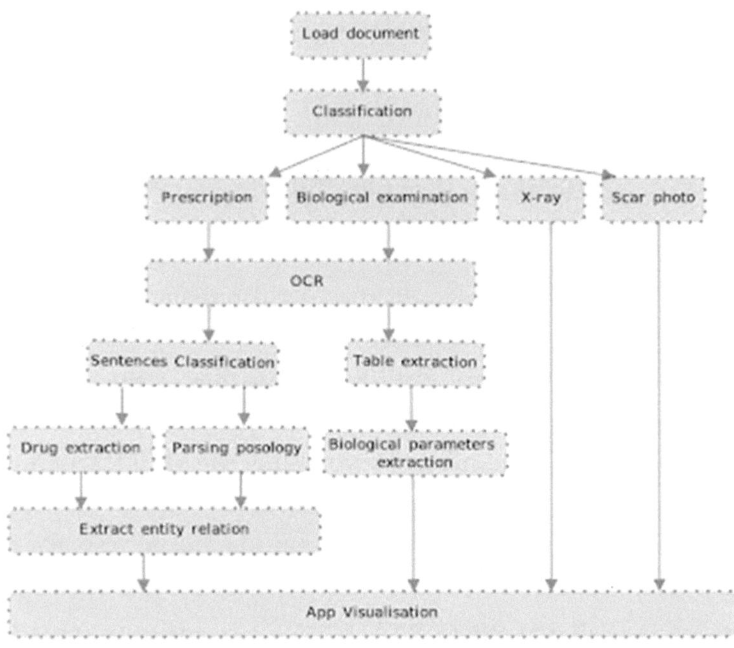

Figure 46: ReLyfe data structuring algorithm

This system starts with the digital image of a page produced by an optical scanner or a digital camera and produces an output JSON file which corresponds to structured data (ICD-10, VI-DAL, HL7, FHIR…) that is more easily interoperable.

This system can be described as shown in Figure 48.

Firstly, we implement the OCR technique to extract text from document in PDF or image format, which include the skew correction. Next, we apply a Convolutional Neural Network (CNN) model to classify the document and associate it to one of four categories (Prescription, Biological Examination, X-Ray, and Scar Photo). Based on the associated category, a new model is applied to the convenient document.

In the case of prescription, we apply the Deep Learning Method from the Spacy Library to classify sentences between Drug, Posology, or Useless Sentences. Depending on the classified sentence, if it is a drug sentence, we apply a particular matcher to find out the drug's name and attach it to a unique ID in the VIDAL databases. Otherwise, a Spacy Rule-Based Matcher is applied to extract the drug-related information (Dosage, Frequency, Duration, Comments) if it is a posology sentence.

Then, we use a Geometric Relationship Approach to assign each posology to its corresponding drug. In the end, we display the result in a Structured User Interface, that is a mobile/web application. In case the document is a biological test results, we extract tables from the document. Then we apply a matcher to collect the existing blood parameters with their associated values and units. In the following sections, a detailed description will be presented for each of the suggested tasks.

a)   **Document Classification**

Before applying Text Analysis to a document, the first step is to separate the text photo from the other type of photo. We use a CNN model as a classifier model to achieve this step to get at the end three classes: Text, Scar, X-Ray. Then, another Logistic Regression Model is trained to separate the text document into Biological Examination, Drug Prescription, and unknown document.

b)   **Optical Character Recognition (OCR)**

In other research works, most projects were operated either on pure medical texts or PDF documents. The quality of documents and how text is extracted were not considered. This implies they had no limitation regarding documents' quality, or the method used to extract text. Despite the limited number of documents used to train our models, there was a diversity in the quality of photos and how the posology was drafted for each drug. Since the extraction of texts is the fundamental step to have clean texts, we did not hesitate to use the service of AWS (Amazon Web Services) to carry out this task. We compared it with other open-source methods trying to get better outcomes but AWS's results were persuasive enough thanks to its performance and detailed text extraction format, which made us keep using it.

This functionality takes as input a document's photo and returns a JSON file containing the text and its Geometric-Related Information in Sentence Level and Word Level.

c)   **Text Pre-Processing**

Due to the low quality of the scanned document, OCR may return unclean text. For this reason, a Data Cleaning move is crucial to make the texts more usable. We apply the following point to the extracted text:
- Removing accents.
- Transform words to lowercase.
- Unify the format of numbers. Remove space between them if they exist.
- Removing the stop words.
- Remove sentences with one word including less than two characters (we got a lot of them).

d)   **Sentence Classification – NER – NLP**

Named Entity Recognition (NER) is an application of Natural Language Processing (NLP) that processes and understands large amounts of unstructured human language. Also known as entity identification, entity chunking and entity extraction.

Before extracting the desired entities from the text, it was more efficient to categorize the text sentences and use exclusively those containing the drug and its information. This step has increased the efficiency of our NER Model since it has made the model focus only on sentences that contain the desired entities. Moreover, with limited databases, training a model to classify the sentence is more realistic and doable than training a NER model.

To accomplish this task, we downloaded 40,000 drug names from the Government Public Drug Database. We also generated 10,000 synthetic sentences that describe how a drug should be taken (these sentences are called Posology).

Moreover, we have produced over 10,000 sentences carrying medical information, patient information, names and all kinds of information that may be present in a prescription other than the drug and the posology.

We trained our classifier using a Bidirectional LSTM Architecture (Long Short-Term Memory). LSTM is an Artificial Recurrent Neural Network (RNN) Architecture used in the field of Deep Learning. Unlike standard feedforward neural networks, LSTM has feedback connections. It can process not only single data points, but also entire sequences of data.

It is used to classify sentences into three categories: Drug, Posology, and Useless Sentences. This classifier achieved an accuracy of 95.23%. The remaining 5% will be automatically ignored by the Drug Extraction Model due to the Rule-Based Approach.

e)   **Drug Detection**

In a French Prescription, the text is structured in a particular way. A Drug is located either in a separate line from the Posology or within the same line. So, after getting the Classified Sentence from the previous model, we will know in advance that there are two choices for the sentence classified as "Drug Sentence": either this sentence contains only the name of the Drug, or it contains both the name of the Drug and its related information (Posology). In addition, generally, between two drug sentences, there is only one or more dosages. We have never seen any information unrelated to a Posology.

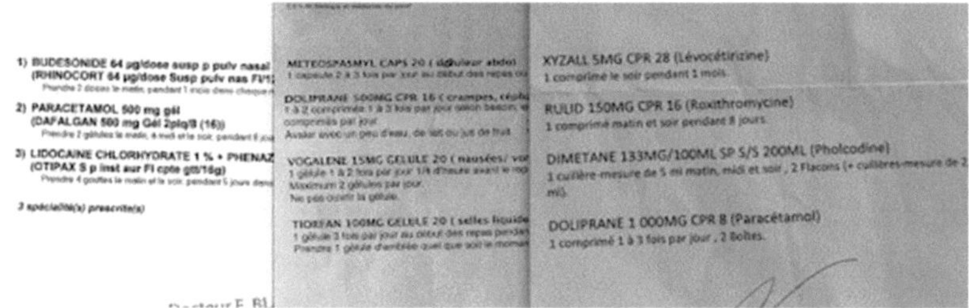

Figure 47: Example of scanned documents

Moreover, one of the main things we are sure about is that Drug names are consistently among the top three words in a sentence. This information led us to minimize the search within the sentence. Hence, we have created a Drug-Matcher relying on a Rule-Based Approach using the Government Drug Databases. Once we have detected the first word of the Drug name, it is used to send a Query to the Vidal Drug Databases and extract a list of all similar names and features. Then, we apply Similarity Measurements to determine the closest and longest contiguous matching sub-sequence to the name in the Prescription.

Indeed, this task is not evident since each Drug is constituted from at least five-word included numbers and units. We can see that clearly in the Figure 47. These Prescriptions were scanned with a smartphone camera. They vary in terms of quality, orientation, and color. Some documents contain the Drug and its equivalent in case it is not available. Our Algorithm should be clever enough to detect this case and choose only one of them. We often come up with the closest despite the difference in word succession or the spaces between numbers and units.

f)   Posology Detection

Like the previous section, after the sentence is classified as a Posology Sentence, a Rule-Based Matcher is applied over the sentence to extract the Related Drug Information. We use the Rule-Based Model from the NLP Spacy Library to create our features matcher. We create four matchers for the four different features that we searched for (Dosage, Frequency, Duration, Comment). Figure 48 shows the rules created for the "Dose Matcher". Our physicians designed more than 100 patterns for each feature. It includes abbreviations, miss-writing, and common mistakes.

```
{"label":"DOSE","pattern":[{"LIKE_NUM": True}, {"LOWER" : {"REGEX":"(graduation[s]?)"}}]}
{"label":"DOSE","pattern":[{"LOWER": {"REGEX":"([\d]amp)"}, '_': {'position_token':True}}]}
{"label":"DOSE","pattern":[{"LIKE_NUM": True}, {"LOWER": {"REGEX":"(ampoule[s]?)"}}]}
{"label":"DOSE","pattern":[{"LOWER": "une"}, {"LOWER": {"REGEX":"(ampoule[s]?)"}}]}
```

Figure 48: Patterns that have developed using the Rule-Based Matching Spacy Library

g)   Drug-Posology Relation Extraction

The AWS "Textract®" API output format includes geometric coordinates of the polygons enclosing the words and the sentences. Based on this information, we created an Algorithm to assign each feature to its corresponding drugs using the geometric features. We relied on human linguistic intuition in this approach. Each Posology is assigned to the closest top Drug while respecting a given distance threshold between their polygons. A Drug can have a Posology composed of several lines.

So, for a given text, if the successive sentences respect the given distance threshold, they are considered in the same section and associated to the same Drug. Otherwise, when the Posology is aligned horizontally with a Drug, it will automatically be assigned to this last one.

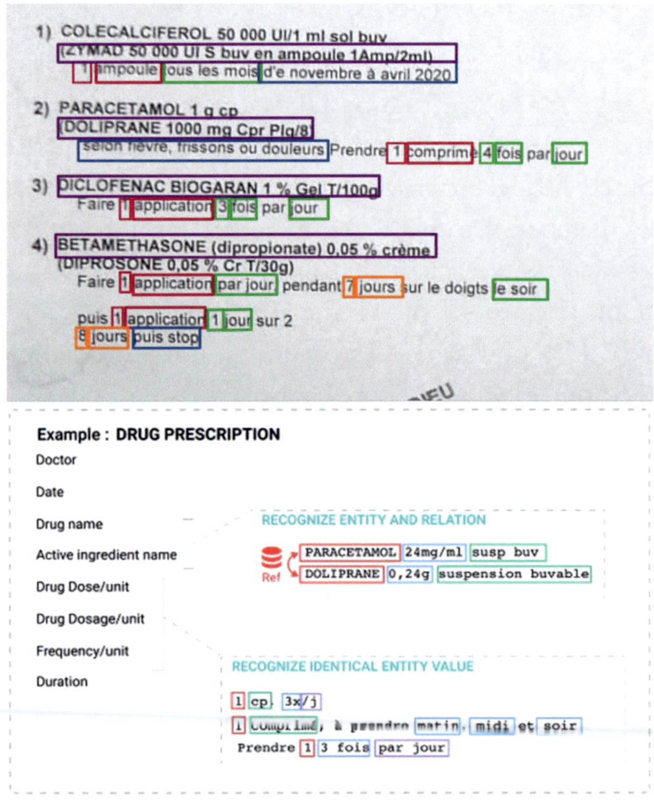

Figure 49: The extracted entities from our approach. We are able to extract the text and apply the relation entity extraction models, even with low quality pictures

h)   **Table Extraction**

Tables are one of the main features in a Biological Analysis document. The tested parameters are always arranged in a tabular format. We have used the AWS analyze text API to extract the tabular shape from the lab results. This table is stored in a JSON file and structured in our databases so it can be used in ReLyfe's future medical prediction research work.

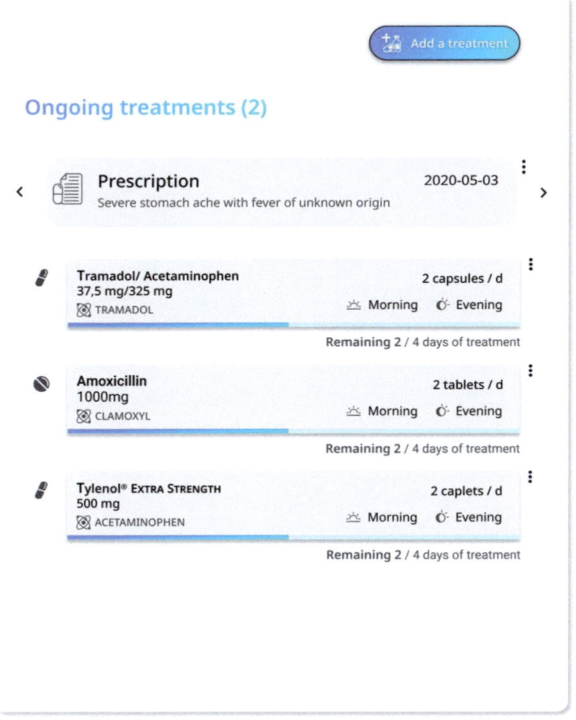

Figure 50: The display of our results in our mobile application after getting the Drug and its related information

i)   **Biological Parameters Extraction**

Matching Models were created to extract existing parameters in a biological examination document.

Each model is designed to detect a specific parameter with its associated value and unit. Sometimes several units are used for the same blood test parameter. However, our models were able to match these other formats and unify them under one standard unit.

An example of this detection can be found in the Figure 50 & Figure 51.

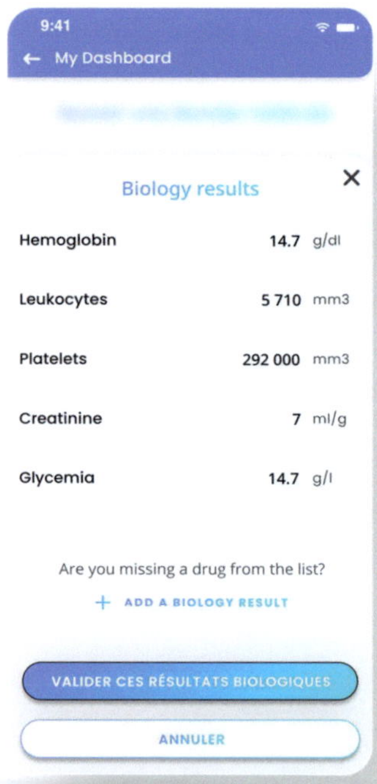

Figure 51: The mobile application display of a structured biological parameters after extracting them by our NER Model

1.14   Legal Aspects

A. Data Anonymization and Encryption

The development of these new information and communication technologies raises many questions regarding Health Data Hosting and Storage.

In compliance with the "Loi de Modernisation du Système de Santé" [Health System Modernization Act] ("LMSS") (France, January 2016), power and control are given to the patient.

Patients must be able to decide whether or not to share access to their data with the healthcare provider they are consulting in person or remotely.

The technology used in this project makes it possible to encrypt and anonymize data.

There is a Dual Security Layer (Hybrid Blockchain-Like Model) with a Public Key and a Signature Link.

The URL generated by entering the Personal Key or scanning the flash-code (heart-shaped code), is a temporary random signature that is generated automatically and instantly (a link that activates a single connection at the time of the consultation and disappears just after the "check" by generating a fingerprint).

Informed electronic consent has been implemented for allowing or denying access to anonymized patient data for medical research purposes.

For this project, we have a Data Protection Officer (DPO) who is responsible for the security of the collected data and compliance with current laws and regulations, in particular the General Data Protection Regulation in Europe (GDPR) and Health Insurance Portability and Accountability Act in USA (HIPAA).

A declaration was made to the "Commission Nationale Informatique et Libertés" [French Data Protection Authority] ("CNIL") under number 2066032v0.

B.   The Security Applied to Health Data

End-to-End Encryption: Data and especially documents in ReLyfe are encrypted, and only the designated patient / health professional has the key to access the actual document.

Firewall: We host the platform on a High-Security Servers certified by the Ministry of Health ("ASIP-Santé" [Shared Healthcare Information Systems Agency] / HDS = Health Data Storage). It has an obligatory firewall. The main objective of a firewall is to control traffic between different trust zones, by filtering the data flows passing through according to defined rules. It is losing its importance, however, as communications are shifting to HTTPS, short-circuiting all filtering.

Anti-DDOS Protection: We have implemented anti-DDOS (Distributed Denial of Service Attack) protection to protect ourselves from denial-of-service attacks.

Anti-Malware: Its objective is to detect and eliminate malicious software in the server.

Access to Data: It is impossible to access the database server data from outside. The database can only be accessed by VPN (Virtual Private Network) and with personal identifiers for access traceability. Only a few people have authorization and identifiers to access the database, particularly for the facilities management required for updates to our ReLyfe application. In all cases, this data remains anonymized.

Two-Factor Authentication: We made it mandatory for users to configure their mobile numbers to activate two-factor authentication on their ReLyfe account. This allows a code to be asked for which is sent by SMS for each log on.

CSRF Token: The platform's forms are protected by a Cross-Site Request Forgery (CSRF) digital token, preventing use of a CSRF vulnerability. A CSRF vulnerability consists in sending a logged-on user a forged HTTP request which points to an action internal to the site, so they perform the action without being aware of it and using their own rights. The user therefore becomes an accomplice of an attack without even knowing it. Since the attack is actioned by the user, many authentication systems are circumvented. The CSRF token prevents this type of attack by generating a token for each form. The controller who receives the form checks that the token sent by the form corresponds to the token generated when the form was created.

Data Anonymization (Figure 52): The database data is anonymized making it impossible to identify which platform user a medical entry belongs to, unless they make this data visible on their Public Emergency Profile, which can be accessed in the event of an emergency, as its name indicates.

Password Hashing: The passwords registered in the database are hashed and concatenated with a Salt-Key using an Algorithm called SHA256 so they cannot be found by a third party who has access to the database.

Protection against SQL injections: We are protected against SQL (Structure Query Language) injections because we use a reputable secure PHP framework that is regularly updated.

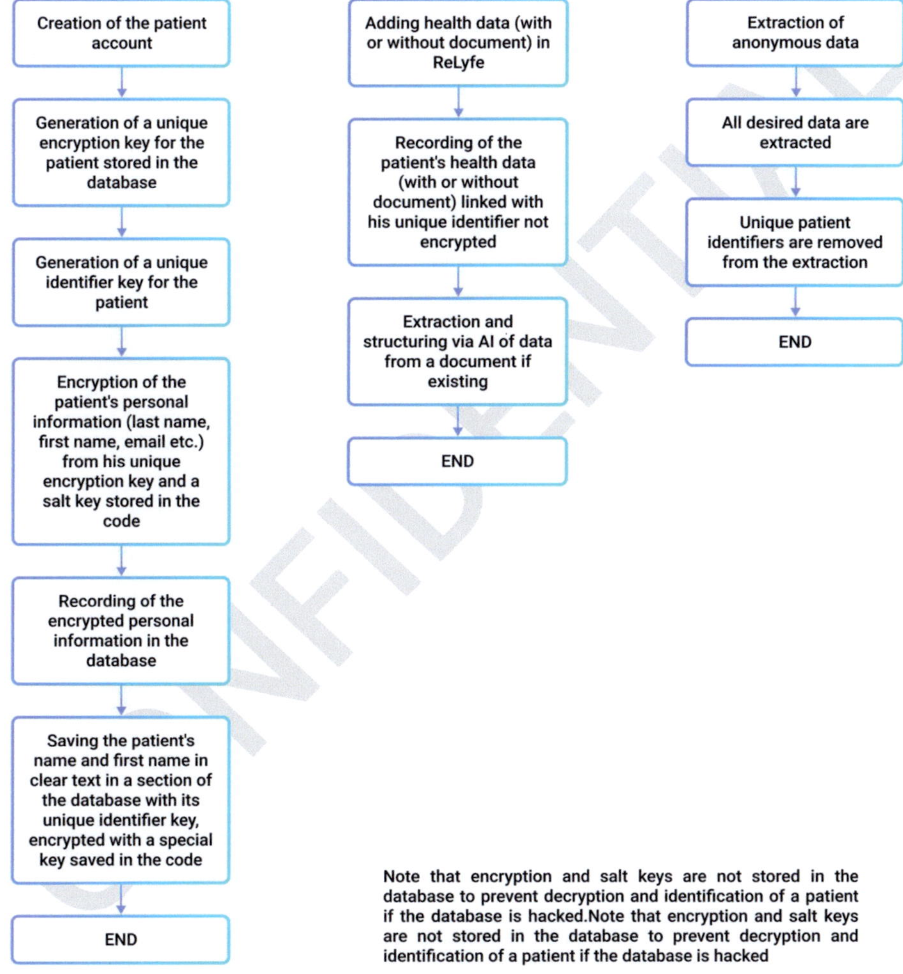

Figure 52: Data anonymization process

We use what are called prepared requests, therefore it is the Database Management System (DBMS) that is tasked with escaping special characters and validating the data entered by the user.

Session Timeout: To prevent a ReLyfe account from being used without a person's consent, sessions time out after a few seconds of inactivity, requiring the user to log on again.

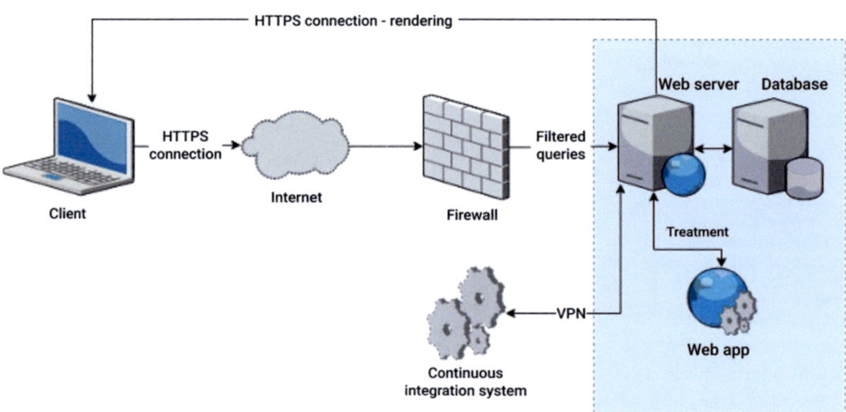

Figure 53: Part of the implemented security process

1.15   Results

A. ReLyfe Mobile App: Creation of a Medical Image Library

The first significant achievement which meets the project's first primary objective relates to information sharing. Let us take the example of photo sharing, one of the built-in functions of ReLyfe PATIENT and ReLyfe PRO mobile applications. It allows photos linked to a disease directly associated with a dermatological problem and/or an operative context to be integrated directly into ReLyfe, for example. Effectively, either the patient photographs, for instance, the progression of a scar via ReLyfe app and directly informs the surgeon who can remotely and instantly see and check it; or the healthcare professional takes photos and enters them in their patient's ReLyfe (Figure 54).

Set against the reality of hospital practice in the Plastic Surgery Department of Tenon Hospital in Paris, and more specifically the challenges and requirements of surgeons and healthcare professionals, the use of this system not only confirmed that the developed technical functions correspond to their expectations, but also helped identify previously undetected improvements to enhance usability.

When this study began, the ReLyfe PRO platform was presented to a surgeon with the aim of helping him improve the efficiency of his practice and facilitating interactions with his patients, with a view to saving administrative time which could instead be dedicated to the doctor-patient relationship.

Already convinced of the benefits of ReLyfe PRO, this doctor quickly made the connection between the functions proposed and his day-to-day practice. Indeed, this practice involves first taking many photos, during consultations and during the pre-operative and post-operative phases, and then creating a scientific research database that can be used much more easily in the future. Generally, medical images are very often exchanged via surgeon's personal telephones and digital applications like WhatsApp!

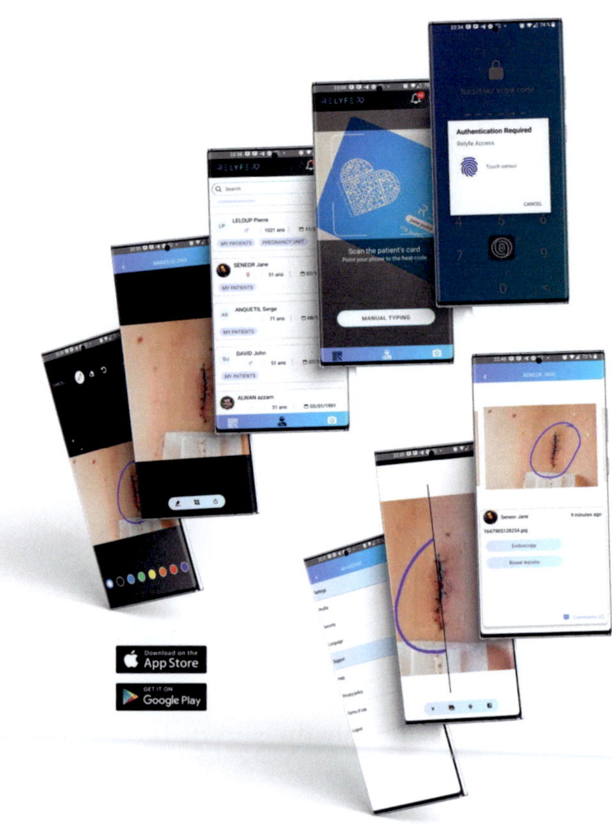

Figure 54: ReLyfe PRO mobile app function where the patient shares the progression of his scar

This practitioner was able to discuss and specify his expectations with the engineers. Plastic Surgery and Dermatology are practices that requires large numbers of photos which are mostly taken directly on the practitioner's smartphone. As they carry out more consultations and procedures, the number of photos increases exponentially. This makes subsequent searches tedious, either for showing the patient the procedure-related developments, for scientific work, for their use in publications or for the preparation of conference materials, all with the patient's consent of course.

ReLyfe PRO mobile app therefore added a labelling tool to the function used to file the photos to each patient, that is based on a Semantic Tree defined with the practitioner according to their specialism. In practical terms, when the practitioner needs to take and store photos, they open the patient's ReLyfe on their smartphone via their ReLyfe PRO application and save the photos, having the option of easily completing fields from the tree with available free fields (simple selection from a menu).
With this in mind, we also built a Search Engine into ReLyfe PRO mobile app so that searches could be carried out by Operation Type, Operation Details, Type of Implantable Medical Device (e.g., Prostheses) and Complication, allowing information to be extracted very quickly whatever the context.

Our work here will contribute to the innovative medical university initiative under way within the Hospitals of Paris, which aims to develop research, university teaching and clinical practice while improving quality of care.

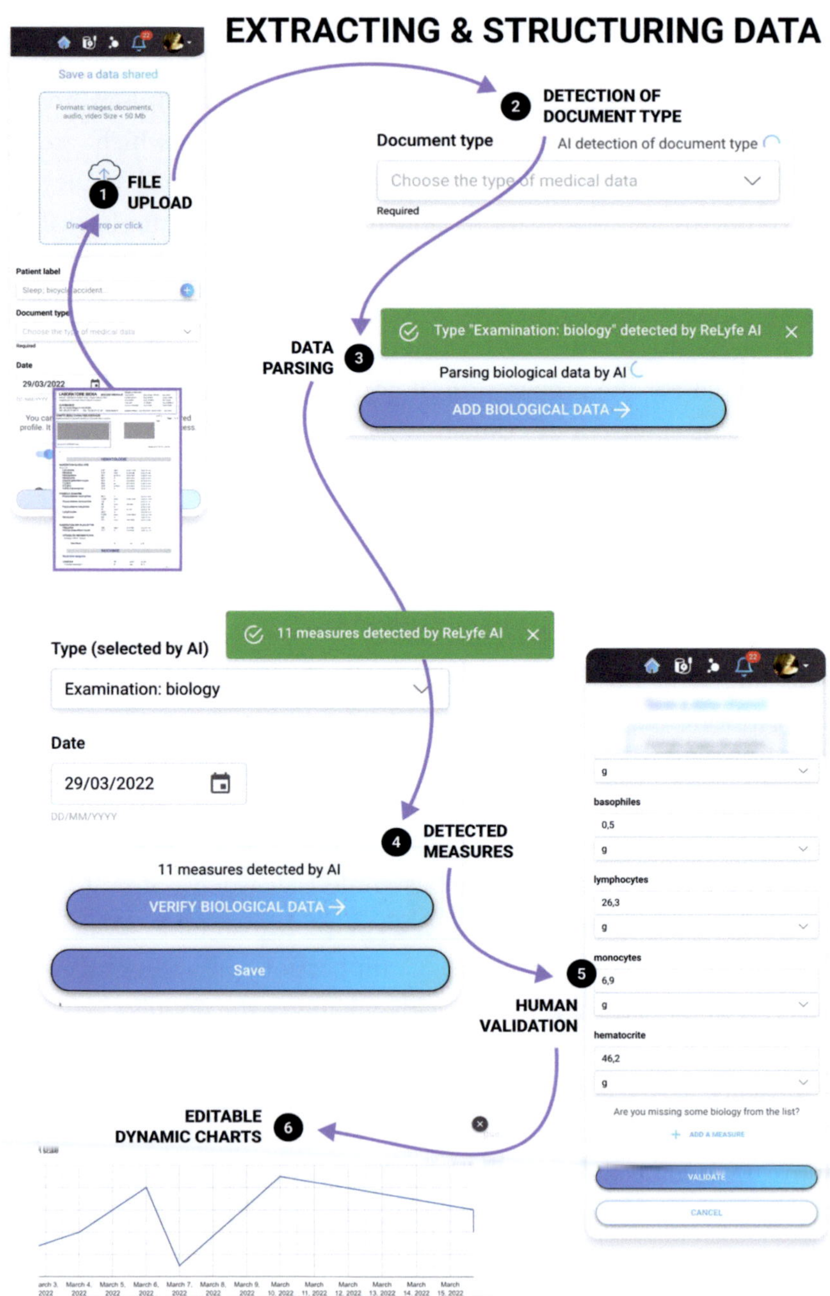

Figure 55: Transition from unstructured files to structured data in ReLyfe

The capability of collecting Patients' Medical Images, directly associated with their Electronic Consent and their Pre-and Post-Operative Questionnaires (Annex 1 and 2) filled in with the expected Score Results, falls within the Medical Universities Departments ("DMU") set up dynamic.

It allows the very fast creation of a Database combined with the production of Collaborative Artificial Intelligence.

After a few months, the system will allow Research Work to progress more quickly and boost Publication Activity which generates revenue for hospital departments, for example.

B. Health Data Structuring

The second significant achievement, which fulfils the second primary objective of this project, related to the technical operational success of transitioning from Unstructured or Semi-Structured Data to Structured Information that is statistically and technologically exploitable (Figure 55).

C. Modified Two-Sided Market Platform Model

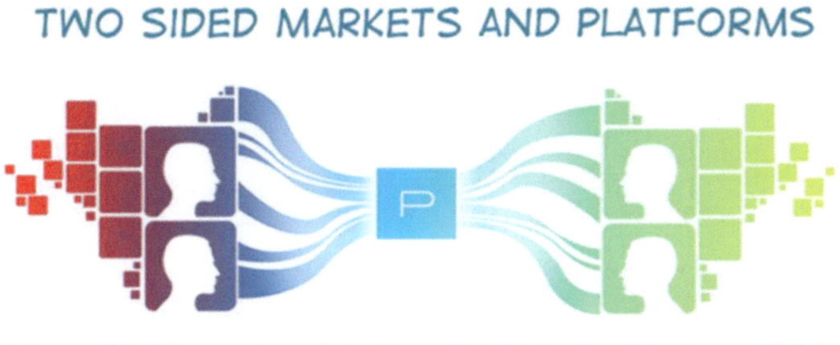

Figure 56: Illustration of the Two-Sided Market Platform (P) Model

One of the secondary objectives of this work, established during the initial development, was to adapt the technology to a suitable viable economic model. Given the universal open-source web platform mode design, the two-sided market platform model emerged as a possible response to this consideration. This model, described by winner of the 2014 French Nobel Prize for Economic Sciences Professor Jean Tirole, is currently used by hundreds of known platforms in several fields on the Internet. The basic element of this model is that of putting two interdependent entities in contact with one another via a Platform P (Figure 56).

The perfect example is social network Facebook. Internet users are free users and do not pay for access, but on the other side of the Platform P (Figure 56), there are professional users who pay for services like advertising.

After scrutinizing and studying this kind of specific market model, I considered it risky and hazardous to apply it as it is to an e-health platform from the outset, given that:
- In this type of model, you need to reach a critical mass of users in the first part to be able to attract users and finance the second part, but we did not want to monetize the data.
- Ethical and Security considerations related to the Protection of Medical Data ("When it's free, you are the product!").

<u>I therefore proposed adapting this market platform model in e-health by applying a new use concept that is both economically and technologically interdependent, but also independent.</u>

1.16   Discussion

In this discussion we will be addressing the example of Kaiser Permanente (KP) which is the oldest and largest non-profit healthcare system in the United States.

Founded in 1945, it currently covers 9.3 million plan members in nine states and is considered one of the most successful.

The organization groups together 167,300 employees, 14,600 healthcare professionals (Doctors, Nurses, Therapists), 37 medical centers and 611 medical offices.

The KP model manages patients according to their Risk Profile, which is presented in the Kaiser Pyramid, allowing the integration of Care Combining Prevention, Primary Care, and Secondary Care.

The system is based on a precise Needs Analysis and Response Scaling according to the Level of Risk faced by the Patient and their Carer:

- <u>Level 0, Healthy Population</u>: Promotion of Prevention and well-being actions.

- <u>Level 1, Low-Risk Chronic Diseases</u>: Self-Care Support, Coordination of the Care Pathway, and the Patient's referral within the health system.

- <u>Level 2, High-Risk Chronic Diseases</u>: Disease Management/Care Management programs aimed at coordinating those involved in the Patient's Care (including the Medical-Social sector).

- <u>Level 3, Very High-Risk and Highly Complex Chronic Diseases</u>: Case Management rationale requiring the Coordination of High-Intensity Care and the intervention of a Complex Case Manager (Figure 57).

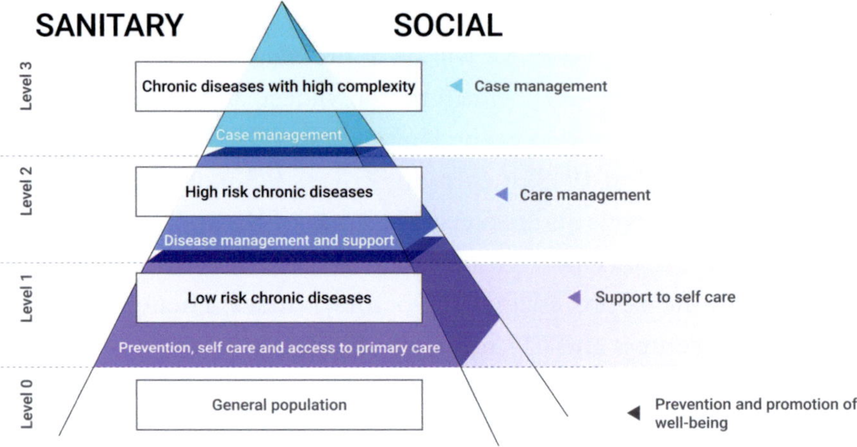

Figure 57: Kaiser Pyramid

In addition to targeting Chronic Diseases, Risk Classification standardizes the Patients' Care Pathway, much like the Coordination applied in the Collaborative Cardiac Care Service for patients suffering from Acute Coronary Syndrome, for example. These patients are monitored by a Nurse who coordinates the care and transition home, and then by Pharmacists who monitor the treatment over the long term.

KP has an innovative information system called HealthConnect®, which allows it to improve its implementation of the Care Pathway founded on the Kaiser Pyramid and achieve concrete clinical outcomes. For example, the Collaborative Cardiac Care Service has reduced the mortality rate of patients suffering from Acute Coronary Syndrome by 76%.

HealthConnect was designed between 2005 and 2008 on the initiative of a group of doctors who wanted access to a Built-in Technology Exchange Platform, combining the two areas, Business and Management of their activity.

Once the KP HealthConnect tool was deployed in the different facilities, Data Analysis was used to structure the organization of the Care Pathway. A set of applications was then developed and is used by the different facilities. The Electronic Medical Records are accessible to all healthcare professionals via Health-Connect on kp.org, the MyHealthManager® Patient Portal is accessible on the Internet or in the form of a mobile application.

All KP members have access to the MyHealthManager portal, which has 4.4 million users and gives patients access to different services.

Each month:
- 2.9 million analysis results are consulted online.
- 1.2 million emails are sent to healthcare professionals.
- 1.2 million medical prescriptions are written online.
- 300,000 medical appointments are made online.

Nonetheless, new challenges now threaten the KP empire, and these challenges are primarily financial. In 2013, KP launched a series of initiatives aimed at lowering costs, in line with the reimbursement restrictions applied by the Patient Protection and Affordable Care Act adopted in the United States in 2010.

One of the most innovative initiatives consists in integrating a scan of the products prescribed to patients into their Electronic Medical Record to allow a Comparative Analysis of the Efficacy of different treatments. This internal benchmark allows the organization to identify the most effective and most profitable treatments, in line with the objectives of the Affordable Care Act aimed at linking reimbursements to treatment outcomes and care.

Moreover, the patients' expectations of the organization are identified via a Systematic Patient Feedback Process integrated into the Change Management Processes.

The main reason for patient dissatisfaction relates to the limitation of KP's territorial logic, and specifically the inadequate exchange of transparent information from one state to another, despite the existence of the Unique Medical Record. Although the organization is integrated into a complete Network, it cannot accommodate Patient Mobility.

Among the youngest patients there is a growing need for Remote Monitoring and Telemedicine media. Young patients are becoming increasingly less inclined to travel to meet a healthcare professional. KP is therefore developing New Care Models to respond to this need, including mobile services.

It has been investing in Predictive Analytics since 2013.

An internal team of 3,000 employees is developing Analyses, Algorithms, and Reports for targeting critical patients.

Moreover, KP is also currently developing Alvin®, a connected car on exhibition in Oakland, California. It is a hybrid car that can be remotely controlled allowing patient examinations to be conducted remotely. The examination of Vital Signs, Blood Pressure and even X-Rays are carried out on board.

The technological challenges therefore lie in improving the use of Data to:
- Create registers of certain Chronic Diseases like Diabetes.
- Compare one patient's situation with that of other patients suffering from the same disease.
- Determine how changes to the Care Pathway can impact Clinical Outcomes.
- Identify the best treatment approaches for patients suffering from several diseases.
- Enhance Expertise and improve the Analysis of Data collected from a patient's first visit to the Emergency Department.
- Develop new innovative tools like Connected Objects.

The health sector requires more Efficient and Secure Systems for managing Patient Medical Records, Pre-Payment Agreements, settling Insurance Records, and implementing and recording other complex transactions, hence the appeal of Re-Lyfe Network (Figure 60) which could provide this sector with the resources it so badly needs.

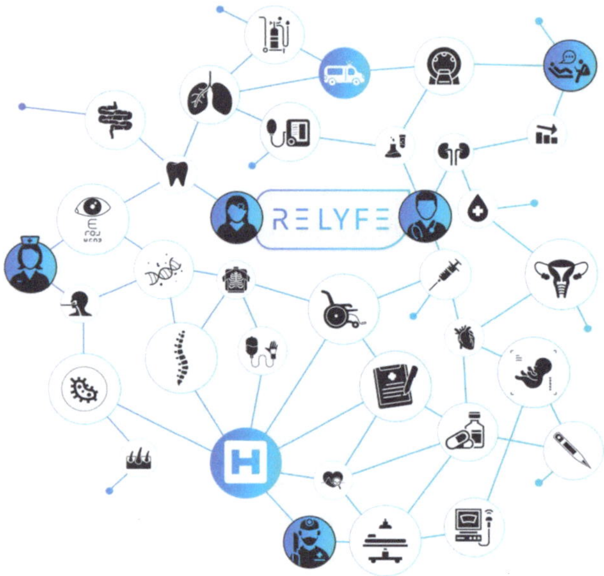

Figure 58: ReLyfe Network

Patient Medical Records are currently managed in Data Centers (with Cloud-type environments), where access is limited to the networks of hospital establishments and healthcare providers. The very costly Centralization of this information makes it vulnerable to security breaches. ReLyfe Network (Figure 58), however, stores the Entire Medical History of each patient with different Levels of Control according to the accessor (Patient, Doctor, Regulatory Organization, Hospital, Insurer, etc.).

It is therefore a secure mechanism that can store and manage a Patient's Complete Medical Profile.

As such, this New Technology is a Hybrid-Cloud Storage medium that is protected against medical history falsification.

It can also reduce insurance case resolution times and improve Efficiency in the production of insurance proposals, for example.

1.17   Conclusion of the ReLyfe Project at this Stage

The development of a Global Intelligent Health Information Management Platform fulfilled the two stated objectives, which were the main barriers encountered in the first study on kidney cancer prediction, i.e., Health Data Sharing and Structuring.

Our technological concept contributes to digitizing the Patient-Doctor Relationship to free up time and increase the Efficiency of communications between the various people involved with and around the patient.

The possibility of having access to Electronic Patient Consent and digitizing Research Protocols will help facilitate health professionals' Scientific Output in real-time, thus advancing Medical Research. Cryptography, particularly its Asymmetric Version, and Network Protocols appear to be interesting technologies for the Secure and Collaborative Management of Medical Data.

However, technological development must not take place without considering the associated economic model. According to my theory, the Two-Sided Platform Model can function in the field of e-health provided it is both economically and technologically interdependent and independent for the two interconnected parties. Technological development alone is not enough to create viable operational platforms.

Virtual Printing built into the Business Software and connected to the Patient' ReLyfe profile provides the platform with unstructured and semi-structured data by extracting information at the source. Our ReLyfe-OCR AI Algorithm can then automate and improve Structuring to make the Data exploitable by selecting information from the ICD-10 database (for diseases) and the VIDAL database (for drugs) (Figure 59).

Our vision and next step are to work on the Clinical Health Data Lake, to detect the gap between an ideal Care Pathway according to the "Haute Autorité de Santé" ("HAS") [French National Authority for Health] or other official worldwide standards and recommendations in Medicine, and the completed and recorded Care Pathway of a Patient in ReLyfe, by collaboratively using our Artificial Intelligence and Deep Learning Advanced Algorithms.

This development is under the guidance of a medical team including myself and a Lead Data Scientist which supplies the Decision Trees to the Machine, so that it can perform Matching with Validated Structured Databases.

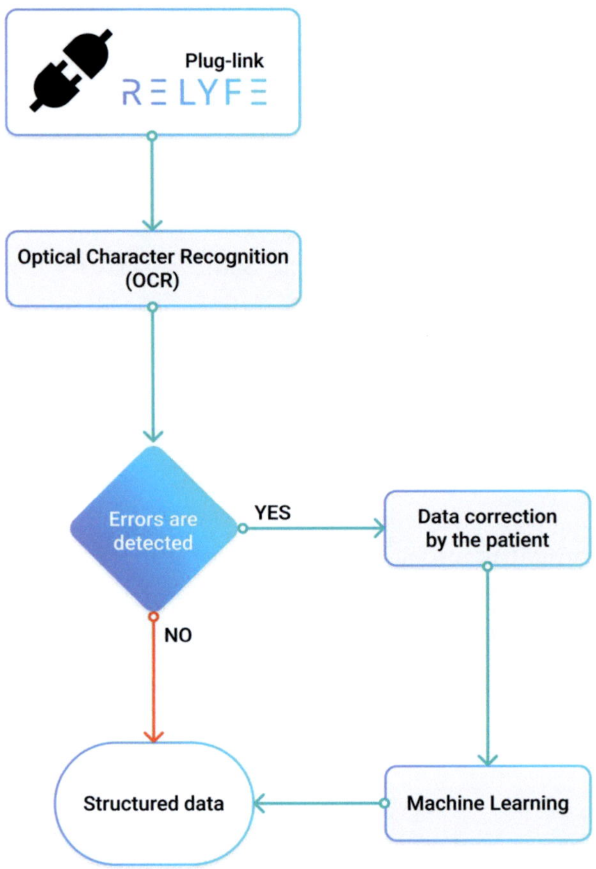

Figure 59: ReLyfe-OCR Algorithm

"A complex issue remains to cover as much as possible all use cases of Patient-Pro exchanges, using the physical aspect of our solution (e.g., card with Heart-Code) for populations whose access to internet or telephony is limited while guaranteeing a secure and private connection difficult to hack. We continue to develop technological bridges to move towards universality and inclusiveness, as health issues concern each of us at some point in our lives. We also need to include voice, assistive technologies and IoT to ensure that no one is forgotten along the way. The development of voice technologies with the translation of structured data, calls and video on the fly would allow for fluid multicultural health exchanges accessible to everyone, wherever they are and in complete autonomy, at a time when medical deserts and conflicts are forcing populations to move."

Quote by Jane Seneor, ReLyfe Head of Product Design

With the development of ReLyfe AI, Health Professionals will have an effective tool for Decision Support and Prevention (Decision Trees from other disciplines, Cross-Referenced Data suggesting an additional examination to be performed, proposal of specialists for a second opinion on a particular case, alerts with comparisons of imagery or monitoring of scars combined with certain specific measures, etc.); and Patients will have the opportunity to be actors of their health, to take control and change certain habits as well as access to exchange with any specialist without geographical constraints or extended professional need.

PART FIVE

OVERVIEW

OVERALL RESULTS

In the first study, the KM applied to the images was used to estimate an Optimal Partition comprised of 8 classes to which the Artificial Intelligence Algorithm randomly attributed colors. Using HES staining of the section, each color was attributed to a given Histological Structure (Anatomopathological Machine Learning, Figure 60).

The interpretation of the Spectral Signatures (Data Mining) between the two M0 and M1 groups identifies two Prognostic Optical Markers. The first belongs to the Tumor and represents a Risk Factor for the onset of Metastases (Cluster 4 Turquoise): OR=2,3 [1,26-4,17].

The second seems to correspond to an Inflammatory Component and represents a Protective Factor (Cluster 2 Blue): OR=0,5 [0,342-0,815].

The other clusters showed no significant results.

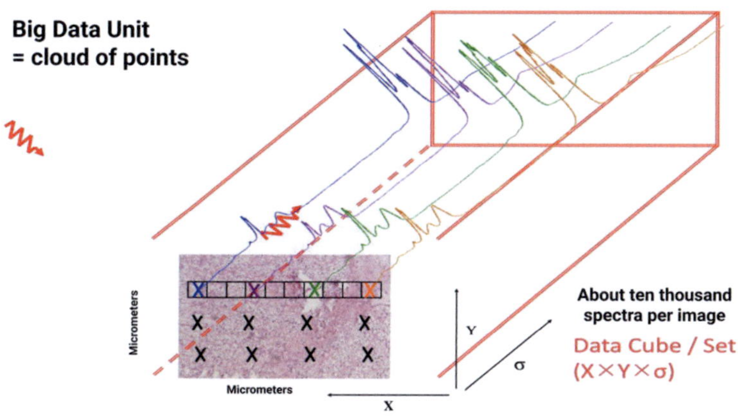

Figure 60: A geometric representation of a Big Data Set

In the second project, ReLyfe.com, a Complete Innovative e-Health Web and Mobile Platform was developed based on the latest Digital Technologies and made securely accessible to Healthcare Professionals and Patients via a card featuring a Universal Unique and Interoperable Digital Identity.

The proposed Hybrid Architecture makes it possible to instantly Share, Structure and Decentralize Information in a technologically and economically redesigned and modified two-sided model (Figure 61).

This new concrete, simple, intuitive, and flexible solution ensures Health Data Portability beyond technical, organizational, or geographic boundaries.

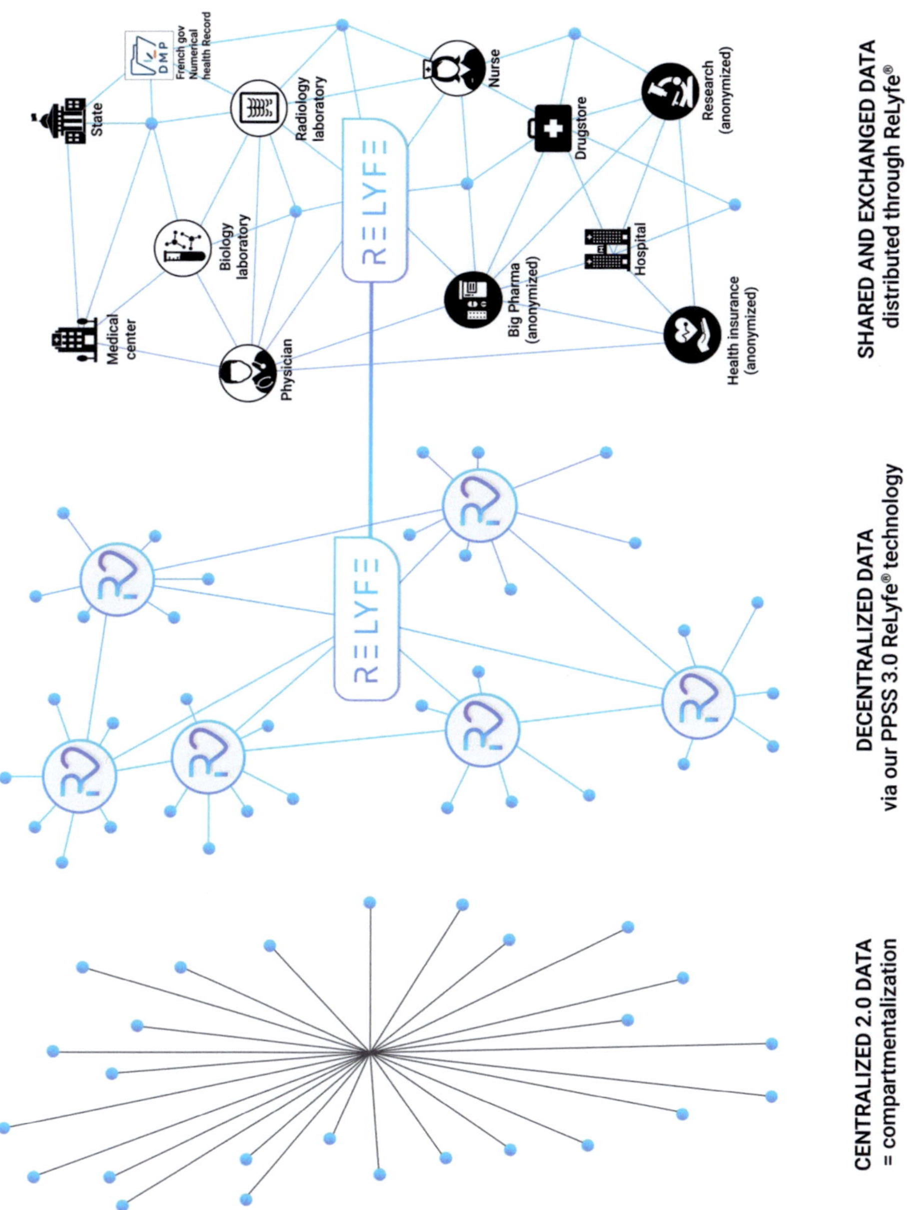

Figure 61: Evolution of the information architecture through the ReLyfe concept

GENERAL DISCUSSION

The first study demonstrates the Predictive Potential of a Big Data Model produced from a small Patient Cohort thanks to the generation of Big Data from spectroscopic images.
However, this Algorithmic Analysis (Figure 62) needs to be validated with Supervised Classification, and training with Deep Learning.

Criteria: contextualize + minimize intra-cluster distance

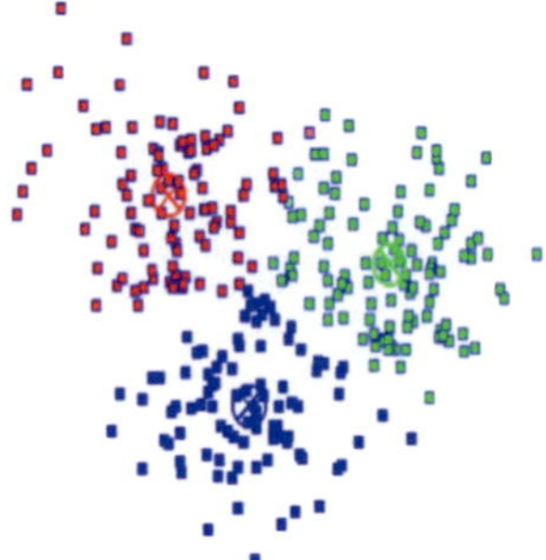

$$\sum_{k=1}^{K}\sum_{s_i \in \Omega_i}\left\|\mathbf{s}_i - \mathbf{v}_k\right\|^2$$

Figure 62: Design of a data cloud algorithmic classification

Although already operational, the ReLyfe model used to create a Real-Time Digital Bridge between Healthcare Professionals and Patients, requires the integration of additional Data, much more worldwide deployments, and long-term application experience, in order to be integrated to standard clinical practices. Economic Impact studies must also be carried out to calculate this Model's Potential to Reduce Public Health Expenditure.

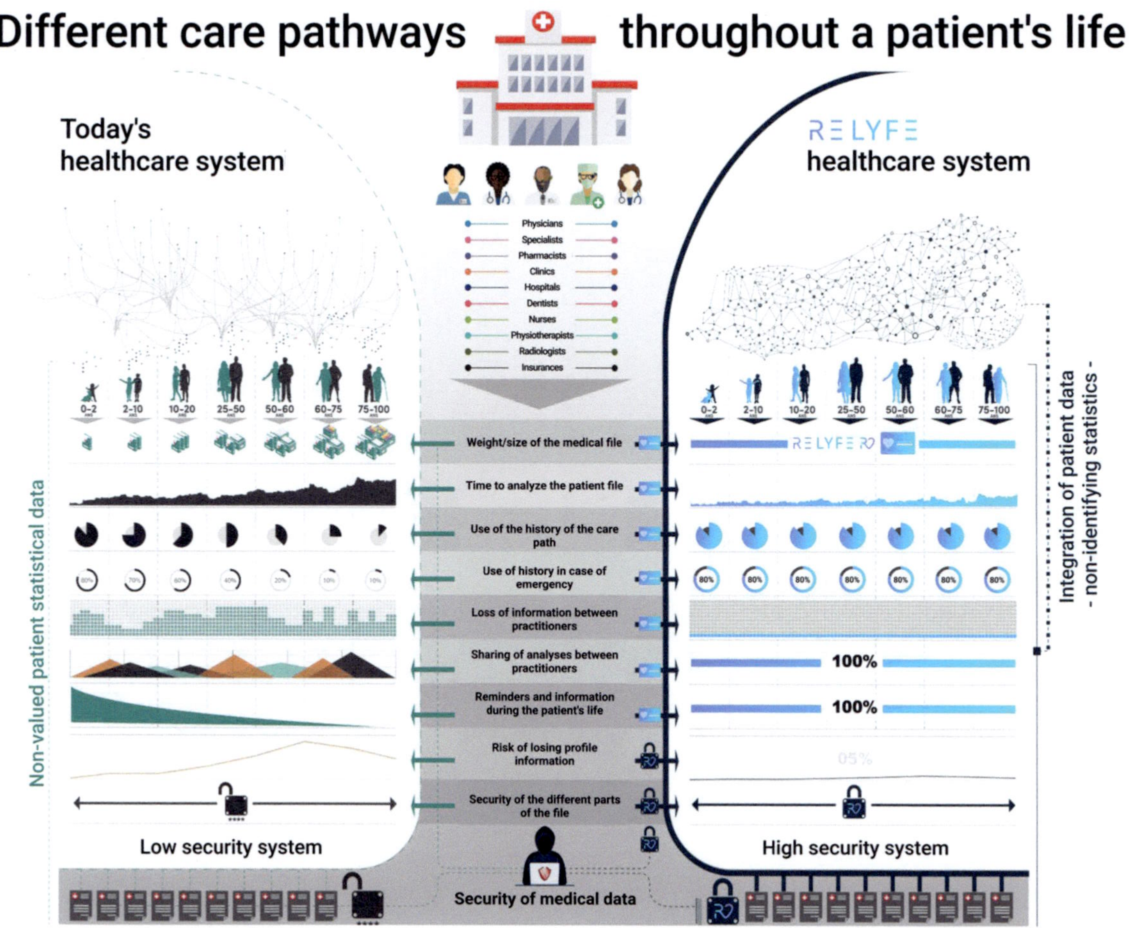

Figure 63: Paradigm shift with a complete data-driven and patient-centered healthcare system

OVERALL CONCLUSION
AND PERSPECTIVES

In any event, this creation could help Streamline the Care Pathway and Prevent any Discontinuity of Patient Care (Figure 63).

Moreover, considering the world's evolving Healthcare Systems, Patient Experience can now be integrated and assessed thanks to our approach, with the incorporation of what is called Value-Based Healthcare, with three notions that seem particularly important for us to consider:

-   PROMS (Patient-Reported Outcome Measures):
    Outcomes.

-   PREMS (Patient-Reported Experience Measures):
    Experience.

-   HRQoL (Health-Related Quality of Life):
    Quality of life.

There is no question that ReLyfe, which can be considered the first Patient-Owned and Patient-Managed Complete Health Software, is moving in the direction of a very popular term: Patient Empowerment.

E-Health and New Digital Technologies can allow more Efficient Sharing and better Structuring of Health Data for Predictive Healthcare (Figure 64).

Artificial Intelligence is not a computer code created at a given moment, but the result of a Learning Process.

The "fuel" of Artificial Intelligence is Data which must be better Shared and better Structured to generate Reliable Exploitable Models.

This work paves the way for a Paradigm Shift with potential future exploitation of Real-Life Health Data, by placing the Patient in the center of a better Coordinated and Connected Care Pathway.

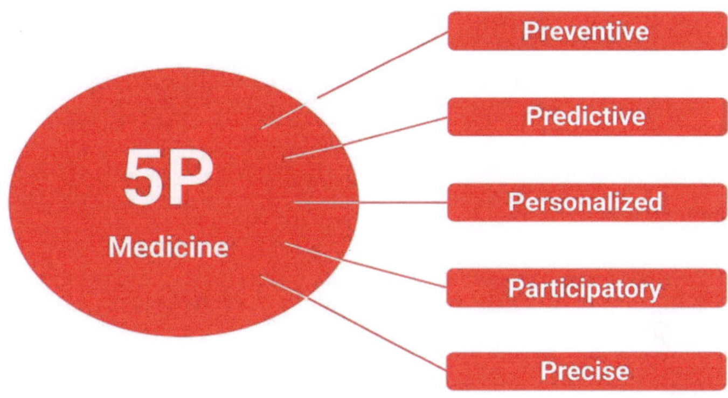

Figure 64: The future of medicine thanks to developments in health informatics

We can also initiate a different way of looking at Health, one that is Less Siloed, more Complete, more Global, more Participative, Collaborative, and Cooperative. All physicians have learned the Decision Trees of the main disciplines and then, caught up in their specialty, no longer have the time to monitor anything other than their specialty. Patients are therefore a sum of specialties which does not facilitate Diagnosis for Rare Diseases or those dependent on multiple connections.

The whole is more than the sum of its parts.

The Covid-19 crisis has taught us that some pathologies are multifactorial, with its Pneumonic and Neurological facets among others, we have gone from Chest X-Rays to MRI to understand the sudden deaths in 24 hours of patients apparently little affected. We rely on the chance of a discovery...

On the Patient side, the world population has expressed its fear of being among the Epsilon cases at risk with this or that vaccine, which has led to a loss of confidence in the recommendations and the notions of Risk/Benefit put forward by Scientists.

With Structured Data coupled with AI and the possibilities of Dynamic Visualization that this combo offers, we could imagine for example another way of perceiving Health through Interactions, Links, Connections, etc.

We would have a clear and ultra-personalized view of Personal Risks, depending on Age, Gender, Environment, Terrain, Personal and Family History Crossed with millions of other individuals and their results in Real-Time. Chronic Diseases Patients could benefit from studies done on groups on the other side of the world.

The Choice will become enlightened thanks to a Personalized and Reassuring Medicine, of which the Patient becomes an actor that he no longer suffers, wherever he is in the world.

On the professional side, one could imagine a Cartography of the body, organs, or measurement results, combined, for example, and weighted or augmented thanks to the Decision Trees of all disciplines and recent Data brought up in Real-World, which would be a robust Decision Aid for any practitioner.

We could also suggest to the General Practitioner additional examinations to be carried out, specialized professionals to ask for a second opinion in one click, suggest recommending his patient to a colleague specialized in the fields having raised an alert, etc.

Medicine will become Preventive First in a Collaborative Way.

We are building an Intelligent System in the form of a Visual Graph, much like ConnectedPapers.com (Figure 65) has changed the way people make Literature Reviews, fill in the gap, search Database which contains hundreds of millions of papers from all fields of Science, have a Visual Understanding of the Trends, Works and Dynamics of each specialized domain.

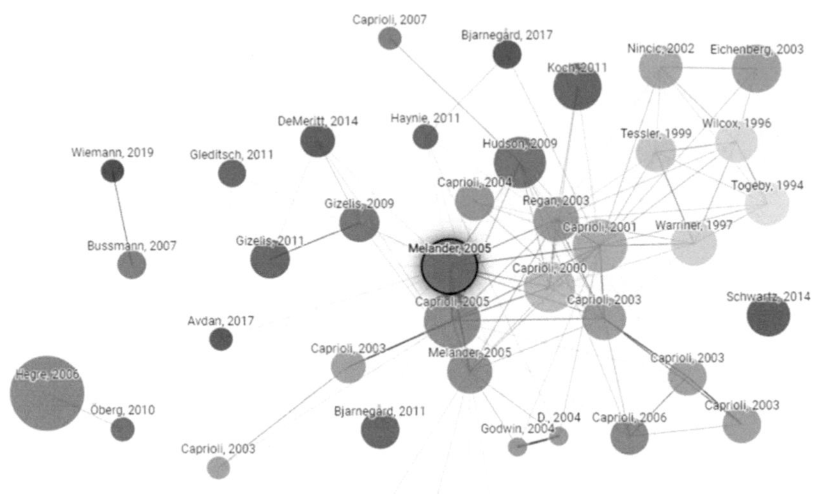

Figure 65: ConnectedPapers Visual Graph

This could trigger a shake-up of fossilized practices and prompt Doctors and Surgeons to innovate, create companies and anticipate the fast-paced development of our professions.

It is also important to adapt initial Medical and Paramedical Training to incorporate these New Technologies into our Basic Learning and everyday practice.

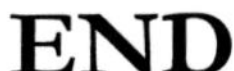

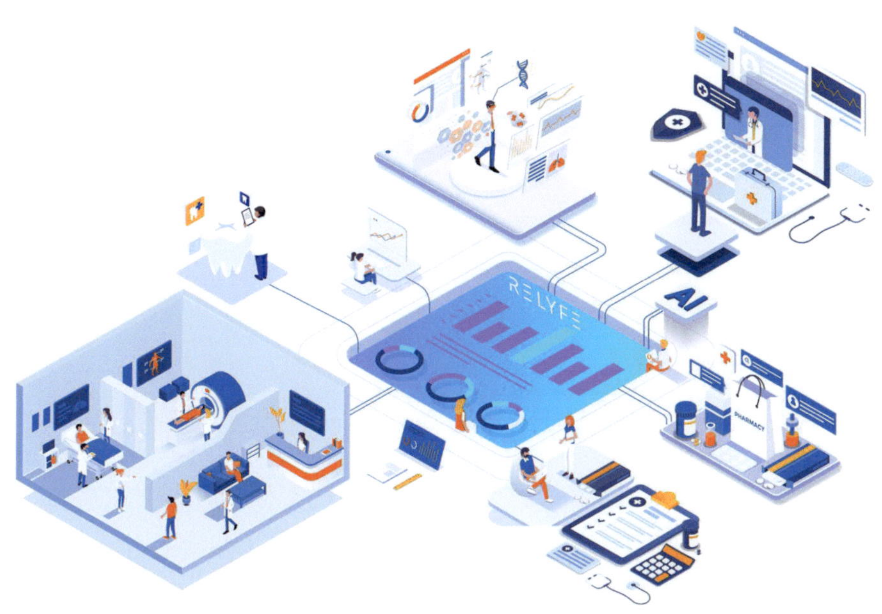

ILLUSTRATION OF A 4.0 CONNECTED GLOBAL HEALTH DATA SYSTEM PROPOSED AND CURRENTLY MARKETED BY THE RELYFE TEAM

THE DREAM, THE IDEA, THE CONCEPT, THE PROJECT, FINALLY BECOME REALITY, AFTER A LOT OF PERSEVERANCE AND DETERMINATION.

TO BE CONTINUED…

"Access to Healthcare must start with Access to Medical Information"
Dr. Adnan El Bakri, Founder and CEO of ReLyfe

King – Man + Woman = Queen…

BIBLIOGRAPHY

1. Yeoh W, Koronios A. Critical Success Factors for Business Intelligence Systems. JCIS. 2010; 50:23-32.
2. O'Carroll PW, Yasnoff WA, Ward ME, Ripp LH, Martin EL, editors. Public Health Informatics and Information Systems. New York: Springer-Verlag; 2003. 792 pp.
3. Mach MA, Abdel-Badeeh MS. Intelligent techniques for business intelligence in healthcare. In: 2010 10th International Conference on Intelligent Systems Design and Applications. Cairo, Egypt: IEEE; 2010. pp. 545-50.
4. Institute for Health Technology Transformation. Transforming Health Care Through Big Data. Strategies for leveraging big data in the health care indusrty [Internet]. [cited the 9 Nov 2019]. Available on: http://c4fd63cb482ce6861463-bc6183f1c18e748a49b87a25911a0555.r93.cf2.rack-cdn.com/iHT2_BigData_2013.pdf
5. Follen M, Castaneda R, Mikelson M, Johnson D, Wilson A, Higuchi K. Implementing health information technology to improve the process of health care delivery: a case study. Say Manag. Aug 2007; 10(4):208-15.
6. Idowu PA. Health Informatics Deployment in Nigeria. [cited 2019 Nov 9]; Available on: https://www.academia.edu/24867442/Health_Informatics_Deployment_in_Nigeria
7. Kirigia JM, Barry SP. Health challenges in Africa and the way forward. Int Arch Med. 18 Dec 2008; 1(1):27.
8. Essoungou A-M. A social media boom begins in Africa [Internet]. [cited 2019 Nov 9]. Available on:

https://www.un.org/africarenewal/magazine/december-2010/social-media-boom-begins-africa

9. Kamadjeu RM, Tapang EM, Moluh RN. Designing and implementing an electronic health record system in primary care practice in sub-Saharan Africa: a case study from Cameroon. Inform Prim Care. 2005; 13(3):179-86.

10. Costa FF. Genomics, Epigenomics and Personalized Medicine. A Bright Future for Drug Development? [Internet]. [cited 2019 Nov 9]. Available on: http://genomicenterprise.com/yahoo_site_admin/assets/docs/Costa_BFE110 9-1.203215611.pdf

11. Raghupathi W, Raghupathi V. An Overview of Health Analytics. Journal of Health & Medical Informatics. Sep 18, 2013; 4(3):1-11.

12. OpinionWay for Swiss Post. The French and connected solutions in health. 2017 Dec

13. Raghupathi W, Raghupathi V. Big data analytics in healthcare: promise and potential. Health Inf Sci Syst. 2014; 2:3.

14. Akinnagbe A, Peiris KDA, Akinloye O. Prospects of Big Data Analytics in Africa Healthcare System. Global Journal of Health Science. 2018; 10(6): p114.

15. De-Graft Aikins A, Marks DF. Health, Disease and Healthcare in Africa. J Health Psychol. May 1, 2007; 12(3):387-402.

16. Okwara D. The state of healthcare in Africa [Internet]. [cited 2019 Nov 9]. Available on: http://www.blog.kpmgafrica.com/state-healthcare-in-africa-report/

17. Unwin N, Setel P, Rashid S, Mugusi F, Mbanya JC, Kitange H, et al. Noncommunicable diseases in sub-Saharan

Africa: where do they feature in the health research agenda? Bull World Health Organ. 2001; 79(10):947-53.

18. UNAIDS. 2012 UNAIDS World AIDS Day Report - Results [Internet]. [cited 2019 Nov 9]. Available on: https://www.unaids.org/en/resources/documents/2012/20121120a_JC2434_WorldAIDSday_results

19. Salathé M, Bengtsson L, Bodnar TJ, Brewer DD, Brownstein JS, Buckee C, et al. Digital epidemiology. PLoS Comput Biol. 2012; 8(7):e1002616.

20. Douek DC, Roederer M, Koup RA. Emerging concepts in the immunopathogenesis of AIDS. Annu Rev Med. 2009; 60:471-84.

21. Young SD, Rivers C, Lewis B. Methods of using real-time social media technologies for detection and remote monitoring of HIV outcomes. Prev Med. June 2014; 63:112-5.

22. Jónasson JO, Deo S, Gallien J. Improving HIV Early Infant Diagnosis Supply Chains in Sub-Saharan Africa: Models and Application to Mozambique. Operations Research. Sep 20, 2017; 65(6):1479-93.

23. CDC. Ebola (Ebola Virus Disease) [Internet]. [cited 2019 Nov 9]. Available on: https://www.cdc.gov/vhf/ebola/history/2014-2016-outbreak/index.html

24. Adepetun A. Africa: Mobile Phone Users in Nigeria, South Africa, Kenya Hit 700 Million [Internet]. [cited 2019 Nov 9]. Available on: https://allafrica.com/stories/201602170661.html

25. Wall M. Ebola: Can big data analytics help contain its spread? [Internet]. [cited 2019 Nov 9]. Available on: https://www.bbc.com/news/business-29617831

26. Anema A, Kluberg S, Wilson K, Hogg RS, Khan K, Hay SI, et al. Digital surveillance for enhanced detection and re-

sponse to outbreaks. Lancet Infect Dis. Nov 2014; 14(11):1035-7.

27. Chang AY, Parrales ME, Jimenez J, Sobieszczyk ME, Hammer SM, Copenhaver DJ, et al. Combining Google Earth and GIS mapping technologies in a dengue surveillance system for developing countries. Int J Health Geogr. Jul 23, 2009; 8:49.

28. Brownstein JS, Freifeld CC. HealthMap: the development of automated real-time internet surveillance for epidemic intelligence. Euro Monitor. 2007 Nov 29;12(11):E071129.5.

29. Bhatnagar A. Web Analytics for Business Intelligence: Beyond Hits and Sessions. Online. Dec 2009; 33(6).

30. Brannon N. Business Intelligence and E-Discovery. Int Prop Technol Law J. Jul 2010; 22(7).

31. Hočevar B, Jaklič J. Assessing Benefits of Business Intelligence Systems – A Case Study. Management: journal of contemporary management issues. 2010 Jun 11; 15(1):87-119.

32. Business Intelligence: The text analysis strategy. In: KMWorld [Internet]. [cited 2019 Nov 9]. Available on: https://www.kmworld.com/Articles/ReadArticle.aspx?ArticleID=18526

33. Glaser J, Stone J. Effective use of business intelligence. Healthc Financ Manage. Feb 2008; 62(2):68-72.

34. Ashrafi N, Kelleher L, Kuilboer J-P. The Impact of Business Intelligence on Healthcare Delivery in the USA. Interdisciplinary Journal of Information, Knowledge, and Management. 9:117-30.

35. Bonney W. Applicability of Business Intelligence in Electronic Health Record. Procedia - Social and Behavioral Sciences. 27 Feb 2013; 73:257-62.

36. Chaudhuri S, Dayal U, Narasayya V. An Overview of Business Intelligence Technology. Common ACM. Aug 2011; 54(8):88–98.
37. Mettler T, Vimarlund V. Understanding business intelligence in the context of healthcare. Health Informatics J. Sep 2009; 15(3):254-64.
38. Yi Q, Hoskins RE, Hillringhouse EA, Sorensen SS, Oberle MW, Fuller SS, et al. Integrating open-source technologies to build low-cost information systems for improved access to public health data. Int J Health Geogr. June 9, 2008;7:29.
39. Deaton A. The Great Escape: health, wealth, and the origins of inequality. Princeton: Princeton University Press; 2013. 377 p.
40. Neal K, De Voe L. When Business Intelligence Equals Business Value [Internet]. [cited 2019 Nov 9]. Available on: http://www.bi-bestpractices.com/view-articles/4744
41. MarketsandMarkets. Healthcare Business Intelligence (BI) Market by Component - Global Forecast to 2023 [Internet]. [cited 2019 Nov 9]. Available on: https://www.marketsandmarkets.com/Market-Reports/healthcare-business-intelligence-market-%20252368925.html
42. Kudyba S, Rader M. Conceptual Factors to Leverage Business Intelligence in Healthcare (Electronic Medical Records, Six Sigma and Workflow Management). Proceedings of the Northeast Business & Economics Association. Jan 2010; 428-30.
43. James J, Versteeg M. Mobile phones in Africa: how much do we really know? Soc Indic Res. Oct 2007; 84(1):117-26.
44. Liu K, Li L, Jiang T, Chen B, Jiang Z, Wang Z, et al. Chinese Public Attention to the Outbreak of Ebola in West

Africa: Evidence from the Online Big Data Platform. Int J Environ Res Public Health. Apr 2016; 13(8).

45. Nsoesie EO, Kluberg SA, Mekaru SR, Majumder MS, Khan K, Hay SI, et al. New digital technologies for the surveillance of infectious diseases at mass gathering events. Clin Microbiol Infect. Feb 2015; 21(2):134-40.

46. Cooper RS, Osotimehin B, Kaufman JS, Forrester T. Disease burden in sub-Saharan Africa: what should we conclude in the absence of data? Lancet. Jan 17, 1998; 351(9097):208-10.

47. Wesolowski A, Eagle N, Tatem AJ, Smith DL, Noor AM, Snow RW, et al. Quantifying the impact of human mobility on malaria. Science. 2012 Oct 12; 338(6104):267-70.

48. Deaton AS, Tortora R. People in sub-Saharan Africa rate their health and health care among the lowest in the world. Health Aff (Millwood). Mar 2015; 34(3):519-27.

49. Freifeld CC, Mandl KD, Reis BY, Brownstein JS. HealthMap: global infectious disease monitoring through automated classification and visualization of Internet media reports. J Am Med Inform Assoc. Apr 2008; 15(2):150-7.

50. OECD. Measuring Aid. 50 Years of DAC Statistics-1961-2011 [Internet]. [cited 2019 Nov 9]. Available on: https://www.oecd.org/dac/stats/documentupload/MeasuringAid50yearsDACStats.pdf

51. WHO. Ebola data and statistics [Internet]. [cited 2019 Nov 13]. Available on: https://apps.who.int/gho/data/view.ebola-sitrep.ebola-summary-latest?lang=en

52. WHO Ebola Response Team, Aylward B, Barboza P, Bawo L, Bertherat E, Bilivogui P, et al. Ebola virus disease

in West Africa--the first 9 months of the epidemic and forward projections. N Engl J Med. Oct 2014; 371(16):1481-95.

53. Patard J-J, Baumert H, Bensalah K, Bernhard J-C, Bigot P, Escudier B, et al. CCAFU Recommendations 2013: Renal cancer. Prog Urol. Nov 2013; 23 Suppl 2:S177-204.

54. Bretheau D, Lechevallier E, de Fromont M, Sault MC, Rampal M, Coulange C. Prognostic value of nuclear grade of renal cell carcinoma. Cancer. 15 Dec 1995;76(12):2543-9.

55. Gaydou V, Polette M, Gobinet C, Kileztky C, Angiboust J-F, Manfait M, et al. Vibrational Analysis of Lung Tumor Cell Lines: Implementation of an Invasiveness Scale Based on the Cell Infrared Signatures. Anal Chem. Jun 2016; 88(17):8459-67.

56. Wolthuis R, Travo A, Nicolet C, Neuville A, Gaub M-P, Guenot D, et al. IR spectral imaging for histopathological characterization of xenografted human colon carcinomas. Anal Chem. 2008 Nov 15; 80(22):8461-9.

57. Tollefson M, Magera J, Sebo T, Cohen J, Drauch A, Maier J, et al. Raman spectral imaging of prostate cancer: can Raman molecular imaging be used to augment standard histopathology? BJU Int. Aug 2010; 106(4):484-8.

58. Nallala J, Piot O, Diebold M-D, Gobinet C, Bouché O, Manfait M, et al. Infrared imaging as a cancer diagnostic tool: introducing a new concept of spectral barcodes for identifying molecular changes in colon tumors. Cytometry A. Mar 2013; 83(3):294-300.

59. Beljebbar A, Bouché O, Diébold MD, Guillou PJ, Palot JP, Eudes D, et al. Identification of Raman spectroscopic markers for the characterization of normal and adenocarci-

nomatous colonic tissues. Crit Rev Oncol Hematol. Dec 2009;72(3):255-64.

60. Crow P, Molckovsky A, Stone N, Uff J, Wilson B, WongKeeSong L-M. Assessment of fiberoptic near-infra-red raman spectroscopy for diagnosis of bladder and prostate cancer. Urology. Jun 2005; 65(6):1126-30.

61. Bensalah K, Fleureau J, Rolland D, Lavastre O, Rioux-Leclercq N, Guillé F, et al. Raman spectroscopy: a novel experimental approach to evaluating renal tumours. Eur Urol. Oct 2010; 58(4):602-8.

62. Crow P, Stone N, Kendall CA, Uff JS, Farmer J a. M, Barr H, et al. The use of Raman spectroscopy to identify and grade prostatic adenocarcinoma in vitro. Br J Cancer. 7 Jul 2003; 89(1):106-8.

63. Bensalah K, Fleureau J, Rolland D, Rioux-Leclercq N, Senhadji L, Lavastre O, et al. Optical spectroscopy: a new approach to assess urological tumors. Prog Urol. Jul 2010; 20(7):477-82.

64. Nguyen TNQ, Jeannesson P, Groh A, Piot O, Guenot D, Gobinet C. Fully unsupervised inter-individual IR spectral histology of paraffinized tissue sections of normal colon. J Biophotonics. 2016; 9(5):521-32.

65. Pakhira MK, Bandyopadhyay S, Maulik U. Validity index for crisp and fuzzy clusters. Pattern Recognition. 2004 Mar 1; 37(3):487-501.

66. Couapel J-P, Senhadji L, Rioux-Leclercq N, Verhoest G, Lavastre O, de Crevoisier R, et al. Optical spectroscopy techniques can accurately distinguish benign and malignant renal tumours. BJU Int. May 2013; 111(6):865-71.

67. Ly E, Cardot-Leccia N, Ortonne J-P, Benchetrit M, Michiels J-F, Manfait M, et al. Histopathological characterization of primary cutaneous melanoma using in-

frared microimaging: a proof-of-concept study. Br J Dermatol. Jun 2010; 162(6):1316-23.

68. Bensalah K, Peswani D, Tuncel A, Raman JD, Zeltser I, Liu H, et al. Optical reflectance spectroscopy to differentiate benign from malignant renal tumors at surgery. Urology. Jan 2009; 73(1):178-81.

69. Hughes C, Brown MD, Clarke NW, Flower KR, Gardner P. Investigating cellular responses to novel chemotherapeutics in renal cell carcinoma using SR-FTIR spectroscopy. Analyst. 2012 Oct 21; 137(20):4720-6.

70. Dagher J, Dugay F, Rioux-Leclercq N, Verhoest G, Oger E, Bensalah K, et al. Cytoplasmic PAR-3 protein expression is associated with adverse prognostic factors in clear cell renal cell carcinoma and independently impacts survival. Hum Pathol. Aug 2014; 45(8):1639-46.

71. International Organization for Standardization (ISO/TC 215). Health informatics — Electronic health record — Definition, scope and context [Internet]. [cited 2019 Nov 9]. Available on: http://www.iso.org/cms/render/live/en/sites/isoorg/contents/data/standard/03/95/39525.html

72. Agrawal R, Grandison T, Johnson C, Kiernan J. Enabling the 21st Century Health Care Information Technology Revolution. Common ACM. Feb 2007; 50(2):34–42.

73. Jung E, Li Q, Mangalampalli A, Greim J, Eskin MS, Housman D, et al. Report Central: quality reporting tool in an electronic health record. AMIA Annu Symp Proc. 2006; 971.

74. Deloitte. Health study 2019: The French and health [Internet]. [cited 2019 Nov 18]. Available on: https://www2.deloitte.com/fr/fr/pages/sante-et-sciences-de-la-vie/articles/barometre-sante.html

75. Deloitte. The satisfaction of the French with the health system is improving, according to the Deloitte Health Barometer (Press Release) – Tout La Veille des acteurs de la Santé [Internet]. [cited 2019 Nov 18]. Available on: https://toute-la.veille-acteurs-sante.fr/123492/la-satisfaction-des-francais-a-legard-du-systeme-de-sante-sameliore-selon-le-barometre-deloitte-communique/

76. CRC Press. Healthcare Informatics: Improving Efficiency and Productivity [Internet]. [cited 2019 Nov 9]. Available on: https://www.crcpress.com/Healthcare-Informatics-Improving-Efficiency-and-Productiv-ity/Kudyba/p/book/9781439809785

77. Smith G, Hippisley-Cox J, Harcourt S, Heaps M, Painter M, Porter A, et al. Developing a national primary care-based early warning system for health protection--a surveillance tool for the future? Analysis of routinely collected data. J Public Health (Oxf). 2007 Mar; 29(1):75-82.

78. Wikipedia [Internet]. [cited 2019 Nov 20]. Available on: https://www.wikipedia.org/

79. Safran C, Bloomrosen M, Hammond WE, Labkoff S, Markel-Fox S, Tang PC, et al. Toward a National Framework for the Secondary Use of Health Data: An American Medical Informatics Association White Paper. J Am Med Inform Assoc. 2007; 14(1):1-9.

80. Baars H, Kemper H-G. Management Support with Structured and Unstructured Data—An Integrated Business Intelligence Framework. Information Systems Management. 2008 Mar 28, 25(2):132-48.

81. Watkins TJ, Haskell RE, Lundberg CB, Brokel JM, Wilson ML, Hardiker N. Terminology use in electronic health records: basic principles. Urol Nurs. Oct 2009; 29(5):321-6.

82. Image: Get out of the frame, imagine new business with blockchain... [Internet]. [cited 2019 Nov 20]. Available on: https://www.google.com/imgres?imgurl=https://thumbor.sd-cdn.fr/e3rO7dlqU5wAlkkoFvZQ1gMM3B8%3D/fit-in/777x550/cdn.sd-cdn.fr/wp-content/uploads/2018/01/Decentralized-Appliction-What-is-it.jpg&imgrefurl=https://siecledigital.fr/2018/01/22/sortez-du-cadre-imaginez-de-nouveaux-business-avec-la-blockchain/&docid=ZDiwLCoEA-L88M&tbnid=Yz_9xxZKA-KKUM:&vet=1&w=777&h=550&source=sh/x/im

83. Dr Adnan EL BAKRI. Do you know the new internet revolution? Will it be enough to save the world (from health)? The "Blockchain" decrypted by Dr. Adnan El Bakri. [Internet]. ® ManagerSante.com. [cited 2019 Nov 20]. Available on: https://managersante.com/2017/11/27/revolution-blockchain-sante-adnanelbakri/

84. Halley EC, Sensmeier J, Brokel JM. Nurses exchanging information: understanding electronic health record standards and interoperability. Urol Nurs. Oct 2009; 29(5):305-13; quiz 314.

85. Reinschmidt J, Francoise A. Business Intelligence Certification Guide [Internet]. [cited 2019 Nov 13]. Available on: http://www.redbooks.ibm.com/pubs/pdfs/redbooks/sg245747.pdf

86. Sahay BS, Ranjan J. Real time business intelligence in supply chain analytics. Information Management & Computer Security. Jan 1, 2008; 16(1):28-48.

87. Loewen E (Liz). Business intelligence: assimilation and outcome measures for the health sector [Internet] [Thesis]. 2017 [cited 2019 Nov 12]. Available on: https://dspace.library.uvic.ca//handle/1828/8882

88. Jordan J, Ellen C. Business need, data and business intelligence. J Digit Asset Manag. Feb 1, 2009; 5(1):10-20.

89. Rochet J-C, Tirole J. Two-sided markets: a progress report. The RAND Journal of Economics. 2006; 37(3):645-67.

90. Rochet J-C, Tirole J. Platform Competition in Two-Sided Markets. Journal of the European Economic Association. 2003 Jun 1; 1(4):990-1029.

91. Giniat EJ. Using business intelligence for competitive advantage: the use of data analytics is emerging as a key discipline for healthcare finance. Healthc Financ Manage. 2011 Sep; 65(9):142.

92. Public Sector Blog | BearingPoint UK. Find the view of our consultants on the issues, the major challenges and the transformations of public services and services to the public [Internet]. [cited 2019 Nov 18]. Available on: https://www.bearingpoint.com/fr-fr/blogs/blog-secteur-public/

93. Teasdale S, Bates D, Kmetik K, Suzewits J, Bainbridge M. Secondary uses of clinical data in primary care. Inform Prim Care. 2007; 15(3):157-66.

94. Wadsworth T, Graves B, Glass S, Harrison AM, Donovan C, Proctor A. Using business intelligence to improve performance. Healthc Financ Manage. Oct 2009; 63(10):68-72.

95. Bonney W. Enabling Factors for Achieving Greater Success in Electronic Medical Record Initiatives. Procedia - Social and Behavioral Sciences. 2013; 73:257-62.

96. Sisense. How Healthcare can tackle changes using Business Intelligence [Internet]. [cited 2019 Nov 9]. Available on: https://www.sisense.com/blog/healthcare-can-tackle-big-changes-using-bi/

97. Coiera E, Westbrook J, Wyatt J. The safety and quality of decision support systems. Yearb Med Inform. 2006;20-5.

98. Fickenscher KM. The New Frontier of Data Mining. Health Manag Technol. 2005; 26(10):26-30.

99. Jee K, Kim G-H. Potentiality of big data in the medical sector: focus on how to reshape the healthcare system. Healthc Inform Res. 2013 Jun; 19(2):79-85.

100. Fosso Wamba S, Akter S, Edwards A, Chopin G, Gnanzou D. How 'big data' can make big impact: Findings from a systematic review and a longitudinal case study. International Journal of Production Economics. Jul 1, 2015; 165:234-46.

101. Financial Times. Data prescription for better healthcare [Internet]. [cited 2019 Nov 9]. Available on: https://www.ft.com/content/55cbca5a-4333-11e2-aa8f-00144feabdc0

102. European leader in diagnostic services. SynLab. [Internet] [cited 2022 March 31]. Available on: https://www.synlab.com/.

103. Explore connected papers in a visual graph. connectedpapers.com. [Internet] [cited: 2022 March 30]. Available on: https://www.connectedpapers.com/.

TABLE OF CONTENTS

INDEX OF FIGURES

INDEX OF TABLES

LIST OF ABBREVIATIONS

AFSA: Armed Forces Security Agency
AI: Artificial Intelligence
AP-HP: Assistance Publique - Hôpitaux de Paris [public hospital system of Paris and its suburbs]
API: Application Programming Interface
APP: Agence de Protection des Programmes [Program Protection Agency]
ASIP-Santé: Agence des Systèmes Informatiques Partagés en Santé [Shared Health Information Systems Agency]
AWS: Amazon Web Services
BI: Business Intelligence
Bpifrance: Banque Publique Française d'Investissement [French pubic investment bank]
CaF: Calcium Fluoride
ccRCC: Clear cell renal cell carcinoma
CHU: Centre Hospitalier Universitaire [University Hospital]
CNN: Convolutional Neural Network
CSRF: Cross-Site Request Forgery
CSS: Cascading Style Sheets
DBMS: Database Management System
DDOS: Distributed Denial Of Service
DMP: Dossier Médical Partagé [Shared Medical Record]
DMU: Département Médico-Universitaire [Medical University Department]
DP : Dossier Pharmaceutique [Pharmaceutical Record]
DPO: Data Protection Officer
EMSC: Extended Multiplicative Signal Correction
EUIPO: European Union Intellectual Property Office
GDPR: General Data Protection Regulation
HES: Hematoxylin-Eosin-Saffron
HDS: Health Data Storage
HIV: Human Immunodeficiency Virus
HTML: HyperText Markup Language

HTTP: HyperText Transfer Protocol

HTTPS: HyperText Transfer Protocol Secured

ICD-10: International Classification of Diseases

IMR: Intelligent Machines Research

InCa: Institut National du Cancer [National Cancer Institute]

INPI: Institut National de la Propriété Industrielle [National Industrial Property Institute]

IoMT: Internet of Medical Things

IoT: Internet of Things

IR: InfraRed

JSON: JavaScript Object Notation

KM: k-Means

KP: Kaiser Permanente

KSI: Keyless Signature Infrastructure

LMSS: Loi de Modernisation du Système de Santé [Health System Modernization Act]

MIT: Massachusetts Institute of Technology

MVC: Model-View-Controller

NGO: Non-Governmental Organization

NICT: New Information and Communication Technologies

NSA: National Security Agency

OCR: Optical Character Recognition

OR: Odds Ratio

ORM: Object Relational Mapping

PBM: Pakhira-Bandyopadhyay-Maulik

PHP: Hypertext PreProcessor

R&D: Research and Development

RCM: Reliability-Centered Maintenance

RCS: Registre du Commerce et des Sociétés [Trade and Companies Register]

REST: Representational State Transfer

RNT: Radical (Total) Nephrectomy

SAS: Société par Actions Simplifiée [Simplified Joint Stock Company]

SGDL: Société des Gens De Lettres [French Authors Society]

SHP: Spectral HistoPathology
SMS: Short Message Service
SQL: Structure Query Language
TMA: Tissue MicroArray
UN: United Nations
URCA : Université de Reims Champagne-Ardenne [Reims Champagne-Ardenne University]
URL: Uniform Resource Locator
USPTO: United States Patent and Trademark Office
UV: UltraViolet
VPN: Virtual Private Network
W3C: World Wide Web Consortium
WebRTC: Web Real-Time Communication
WHO: World Health Organization
WWW: World Wide Web
XML: Extensible Markup Language

BREAST-Q™
AUGMENTATION MODULE (PRE-OPERATIVE) 1.0

The questions below relate to your breasts. In the last two weeks, have you felt:

		Never	Rarely	Some-times	Often	All the time
a.	Confident in society?	1	2	3	4	5
b.	Happy with yourself?	1	2	3	4	5
c.	Confident in your clothes?	1	2	3	4	5
d.	Equal to other women?	1	2	3	4	5
e.	Attractive?	1	2	3	4	5
f.	Comfortable with your body?	1	2	3	4	5
g.	Self-confident?	1	2	3	4	5
h.	Confident about your body?	1	2	3	4	5
i.	Confident?	1	2	3	4	5

In the last two weeks, have you had:

		Never	Rarely	Some-times	Often	All the time
a.	Pain in your breasts?	1	2	3	4	5
b.	A feeling of hardness in your breasts?	1	2	3	4	5
c.	Difficulty lifting heavy objects?	1	2	3	4	5
d.	Difficulty carrying out an intense physical activity (e.g. running or sport)?	1	2	3	4	5
e.	Difficulty lifting or moving your arms?	1	2	3	4	5

The questions below relate to your sex life. In general, do you feel:

	Never	Rarely	Some-times	Often	All the time	Not re-levant
a. Sexually desirable when you are <u>dressed</u>?	1	2	3	4	5	NR
b. At ease during your sexual relations?	1	2	3	4	5	NR
c. Sexually self-confident?	1	2	3	4	5	NR
d. Sexually attractive when you are <u>naked</u>?	1	2	3	4	5	NR
e. Sexually self-confident with regard to the appearance of your breast(s) when you are <u>naked</u>?	1	2	3	4	5	NR

BREAST-Q™
AUGMENTATION MODULE (POST-OPERATIVE)
1.0

The questions below relate to your breasts. In the last two weeks, have you been <u>satisfied or not</u>:

		Not at all satisfied	Not very satisfied	Quite satisfied	Very satisfied
a.	With your reflection in the mirror when you are <u>dressed</u>?	1	2	3	4
b.	With the balance between the size of your breasts and the rest of your body?	1	2	3	4
c.	With the fit of your bra?	1	2	3	4
d.	With the depth of your cleavage when you wear a bra?	1	2	3	4
e.	With the size of your re-constructed breast(s)?	1	2	3	4
f.	With your reflection in the mirror when you are <u>naked</u>?	1	2	3	4

POSTFACE

This book introduces a worldwide revolutionary concept, patented, invented and directed by Dr. Adnan El Bakri. It is the result of 18 years of study, research and development, with a lot of hard work, perseverance, sacrifices and sleepless nights. He has spent literally half of his life on it, he is now the 35 years old Founder and CEO of ReLyfe Group, officially supported by the Ministry of Innovation and Research, and financially backed by the French Public Investment Bank.

French-Lebanese physician, entrepreneur, surgeon, scientist, researcher in Artificial Intelligence and digital health expert, he graduated from the Faculties of Medicine of Marseille and Reims, and from the Universities of Aix-en-Provence, URCA and Paris-Saclay. Born in an underprivileged neighborhood in Lebanon, from poor parents, he suffered during his childhood from the difficulty of access to healthcare, so he made it his fight. In 2004 he left his family and arrived in France at the age of 17 with no money. Homeless, he slept for the first months in the corridors of the Faculty of La Timone. In 2016, he was naturalized on merit by the President of the Republic and then medaled with Palm of the Universal League of Public Good, member of the UN, with decoration of the Republican Guard in 2019. He became trilingual (English, French, Arabic).

Pioneer of e-health in France, he was VP of the National Council of Young Surgeons and then founded the National Council of E-Health, he was also member of the Board of E-Health World in Monaco. He created with his team the first private, interactive, interoperable and international AI-powered Care Pathway belonging to the patient, within a unique timeline, Medical Collaboration Platform, linking any health professional in the world, easily, in several languages, on ReLyfe.com

Multi-awarded with 13 official distinctions, his work has been recognized by the National Academy of Surgery and presented at conferences around the world where he introduced and developed a new dynamic rule-based AI model for structuring a global health data lake in real-time to move medicine towards the 5Ps (Prevention, Prediction, Participation, Precision, Proof) by involving patients. He invented the first Virtual Printer that easily and instantly connects medical information exchanges between health professionals and patients in a universal and secure way, regardless of the software or device used, reducing carbon footprint. He has proposed an adaptation of the two-sided market economic model described by the French Nobel Prize in Economics, Prof. Jean Tirole, to e-health. He has produced or participated in more than twenty publications. In 2017, he was in charge of writing the program on the future of the French healthcare system for one of the candidates for the Presidency of the Republic where he highlights a sclerotic bureaucracy and a considerable technological gap. He is one of the first doctors to talk about Value-Based Healthcare and PROMS/PREMS. He advocates a paradigm shift for a broader, collaborative and prospective EBM (Evidence-Based Medicine), with smart technological support for medical decisions in network mode, coupled with social and ethical values. He has been voted best entrepreneur of the year.

In 2021, he is selected in the prestigious Choiseul Institute ranking among the most promising young talents and business leaders, describing him as a pure product of the meritocracy.

Despite all the difficulties, he single-handedly succeeded in raising $10 million in seed money and transforming his invention into a company and then into a marketed product, in one of the most complex fields and context. His project is now being developed in Europe, Africa, Canada, USA and Middle East. He has always sought to have the most positive impact and to change the world.

www.adnanelbakri.com

HIPPOCRATIC OATH

In the presence of the Masters of this Faculty, my fellow students and in accordance with the Hippocratic tradition, within my practice in the medical profession, I promise and swear that at all times I shall act honorably and with integrity.

I shall give free care to the indigent and shall never demand to be paid more than my work deserves.

In entering people's homes, I shall treat their private affairs confidentially and shall not attempt to corrupt or seduce.

With respect and gratitude to my Masters, I will pass on to their children the instruction I have received from their fathers.

May my fellow men and fellow doctors grant me their respect if I remain true to my promises.

May I be dishonored and scorned if I transgress them.

Don't be discouraged, it's often the last key in the bunch
that opens the lock.